CARDIAC SARCOIDOSIS

Collected Reprints (1977-2019)

By

William C. Roberts, MD

and

Colleagues

ISBN: 979-8-88680-088-3
Printed in the United States of America on acid-free paper.

Preface

Sarcoidosis, a systemic disease, can affect virtually any body organ, including the heart. If sarcoid in the heart causes cardiac dysfunction, it spares dysfunction of the body's non-heart organs. That is an important principle of cardiac sarcoidosis. The condition either goes down the cardiac road, sparing the non-cardiac organs, or it goes down the noncardiac road, sparing the heart.

Sarcoidosis has always been defined by the presence of giant-cell granulomas in one or more body organs. The granulomas also contain many lymphocytes, but cardiac sarcoidosis may occur in hearts with multifocal scars in the absence of granulomas. The hearts with and without granulomas are similar, characterized grossly by multifocal scars in the ventricular walls, often involving only the subepicardial portions, and sparing the atrial walls. The findings are unique to cardiac sarcoidosis. These hearts with multifocal ventricular scars without granulomas have been referred to as "burnt-out sarcoidosis." These gross cardiac features are unique for sarcoidosis. The epicardial coronary arteries are not narrowed. Both ventricular cavities are very dilated.

Diagnosis of cardiac sarcoidosis clinically is often difficult. Most of these patients come to heart transplantation with a clinical diagnosis of "idiopathic dilated cardiomyopathy." Since the granulomas are focal, myocardial biopsy is a hit-or-miss procedure. The electrocardiogram usually shows low QRS voltage.

—William C. Roberts, MD

Table of Contents

*Articles are numbered based on WCR's CV.

Sarcoidosis of the Heart

A Clinicopathologic Study of 35 Necropsy Patients (Group I) and Review of 78 Previously Described Necropsy Patients (Group II)

WILLIAM C. ROBERTS, M.D.
Bethesda, Maryland

HUGH A. McALLISTER, Jr., M.D.
Washington, D.C.

VICTOR J. FERRANS, M.D., Ph.D.
Bethesda, Maryland

From the Pathology Branch, National Heart, Lung and Blood Institute, National Insitutes of Health, Bethesda, Maryland; and the Cardiovascular Department, Armed Forces Institute of Pathology, Washington, D.C. Requests for reprints should be addressed to Dr. William C. Roberts, Building 10A, Room 3E-30, National Institutes of Health, Bethesda, Maryland 20014. Manuscript accepted October 6, 1976.

Certain clinical and morphologic observations are described in 35 necropsy patients with cardiac sarcoidosis (group IA and IB), and similar observations are summarized in 78 previously described necropsy patients with cardiac sarcoidosis (group IIA and IIB). All patients had non-necrotic ("hard") granulomas in lymph nodes and either sarcoid granulomas in the heart (108 patients) or transmural myocardial scarring (five patients) unassociated with coronary arterial narrowing, i.e., healed granulomas. The 113 patients (groups I and II) whose data are analyzed also were divided into those in whom cardiac dysfunction clearly was the result of sarcoid granulomatous infiltration of the heart (89 patients) (groups IA and IIA), and those in whom cardiac dysfunction, if present, was clearly not the result of sarcoid involvement of the heart (24 patients) (groups IB and IIB).

Analysis of the 89 patients in groups IA and IIA disclosed that death was *sudden* (arrhythmia) in 60 (67 per cent), secondary to progressive *congestive cardiac failure* in 20 (23 per cent), from *recurring pericardial effusion* in three (3 per cent) and from other or unknown causes in six (7 per cent). Sudden death was the initial manifestation of sarcoidosis in 10 (17 per cent) of the 60 patients who died suddenly. Other than premature ventricular beats, *ventricular tachycardia* was the most common arrhythmia (17 patients), and *complete heart block* was the most common conduction disturbance (25 patients). *Complete bundle branch block* occurred in 21 patients. *Ventricular aneurysm* (eight patients) and *papillary muscle dysfunction* (possibly 16 patients) were other cardiac disturbances observed.

Although *corticosteroid therapy* tends to cause fibrous replacement of myocardial sarcoid granulomas, a possible consequence of this medication is the development of ventricular aneurysm.

Most patients with cardiac sarcoidosis causing dysfunction (groups IA and IIA) presented initially with manifestations related to the heart. Furthermore, most patients with cardiac sarcoidosis have little or no clinical evidence of dysfunction of an organ system other than the heart. Usually the course in patients with extensive cardiac sarcoidosis is not prolonged.

Sarcoidosis, a systemic granulomatous disease of undetermined etiology and pathogenesis, most often involves lymph nodes, lungs, liver, spleen, skin, eyes, phalangeal bones and parotid glands, but other organs and tissues also may be affected. Cardiac involvement in patients with sarcoidosis has been reported on many occasions, but most reports are isolated case studies. The present study is a clinicopathologic analysis of a relatively large number of necropsy patients with cardiac sarcoidosis. It focuses on the varying types of functional and morphologic cardiac alterations in patients with cardiac sarcoidosis and, in addition, summarizes previous reports of this condition.

METHODS

The data on all the necropsy patients having cardiac sarcoidosis studied in the Pathology Branch, National Heart, Lung and Blood Institute, and in the Cardiovascular Registry of the Armed Forces Institute of Pathology are included in this analysis. A total of 35 patients was available for study (groups IA and IB). Prerequisites for inclusion in this study included (1) the presence of sarcoid-type, i.e., "hard" (non-necrotic) granulomas in lymph nodes, and (2) either the presence of sarcoid-type granulomas in the heart or the presence of transmural myocardial scarring unassociated with significant luminal narrowing of the extramural coronary arteries. The clinical and necropsy records, and the histologic sections from all body organs were reviewed. Excluding the one patient in whom the atrioventricular node and bundle were serially sectioned (sections cut a thickness of 6 μ and every fifth section was stained by hematoxylin and eosin), a total of 230 histologic sections of heart were examined, an average of six per patient (range one to 20). At least one histologic section of left ventricle was examined in every patient. Sections of other portions of the heart were available for reexamination in 31 patients: these included the ventricular septum (27 patients), the right ventricular free wall (25 patients), the right atrial wall (16 patients) and the left atrial wall (14 patients). The autopsy protocols also were examined for information regarding the presence or absence of granulomas in the various portions of the heart. Information was obtained regarding the presence or absence of sarcoid-type granulomas in lymph nodes (all patients) and lung, liver, and spleen (32 patients). Weights of the heart were available in 30 patients, and of the spleen, liver and both lungs in each of 20 patients. The available clinical information was examined in all 35 patients. Similar information was obtained on previously described cases of cardiac sarcoidosis. The classification used to group the 35 personally studied patients and the 78 previously described cases of cardiac sarcoidosis is outlined in Table I.

RESULTS

Certain clinical and morphologic observations in the 35 personally studied patients (groups IA and IB) are summarized in Tables II and III. For analysis of the cardiac disturbances, the 35 patients were subdivided into those in whom cardiac dysfunction clearly was the result of sarcoid granulomatous infiltration of the heart (26 patients, group IA, Table II), and those in whom cardiac dysfunction, if present, was clearly not the result of sarcoid granulomatous infiltration of the heart (nine patients, group IB, Table III).

At necropsy, 25 of these 26 patients (group IA) had grossly visible, usually large, granulomas in their hearts; the remaining patient had transmural myocardial scars unassociated with significant coronary arterial luminal narrowing. The other nine patients (group IB) were subdivided according to their predominant clinical features as shown in Table III. All nine of these patients had sarcoid granulomas in their hearts, but these granulomas were small; in eight patients they were visible only by histologic examination. This report focuses primarily on the 26 patients with cardiac dysfunction clearly secondary to sarcoid infiltration of the heart (group IA).

Observations in the Patients with Cardiac Dysfunction Secondary to Cardiac Sarcoidosis (Group IA). Cardiac dysfunction in the 26 patients in whom it was caused by cardiac sarcoidosis was variously manifested by arrhythmias and conduction disturbances, congestive cardiac failure and recurring pericardial effusions (Table II). These cardiac disturbances accounted for death in 25 of the 26 patients.

Arrhythmias or **conduction disturbances,** or both, were documented in 16 of these patients; electrocar-

TABLE I Cardiac Sarcoidosis: Necropsy Patients Analyzed

	Totals	Causing Cardiac Dysfunction (Subgroup A)		Not Causing Cardiac Dysfunction (Subgroup B)	
		No.	%	No.	%
Personally studied patients (group I)	35	26	74	9	26
Previously described patients (group II)	78	63	81	15	19
Totals	113	89	79	24	21

diograms were never recorded in six of the remaining 10 patients. Episodes of **ventricular tachycardia** were documented by electrocardiogram in five patients; 12 patients had ventricular premature beats. Four patients, two of whom also had episodes of ventricular tachycardia, had **atrial arrhythmias:** atrial fibrillation in two, atrial tachycardia in one and frequent atrial premature beats in one.

Heart block was confirmed by electrocardiogram in seven patients: prolongation of the P-R interval in one patient and complete heart block in six. In five of them the third degree heart block was present from two to six months; in the sixth patient it appeared about 2 hours before death. Three of the five patients with long-term complete heart block had syncope, which was the initial manifestation of sarcoidosis in each of them. Among the five patients with long-term complete heart block, the conduction disturbance, once it appeared, was persistent thereafter in four and periodic in one. In the latter patient, fibrous scarring associated with lymphocytic-cell infiltration was present at necropsy in the most cephalad portion of the muscular ventricular septum, whereas in the four patients with permanent complete heart block, large granulomas were still

TABLE II Cardiac Sarcoidosis Causing Cardiac Dysfunction: Clinical and Morphologic Observations in 26 Personally Studied Patients (Group IA)

	Mode of Death				
	Sudden	Congestive Heart Failure	Pericardial Effusion	Noncardiac	Totals
Patients (no.)	17	6	2	1	26
Age (yr)					
Range	21–74	26–73	35–47	34	21–74
Average	36	51	41	34	40
Race					
Black	9	3	2	0	14 (54)
White	7	2	0	1	10 (38)
Unknown or other	1	1	0	0	2 (8)
Sex					
Male	10	2	1	1	14 (54)
Female	7	4	1	0	12 (46)
Duration of symptoms (mo)					
Range	0–53	1–18	16, 18	48	0–53
Average	9*	7	17	48	11
Atrial arrhythmia	3	1	0	0	4 (15)
Ventricular premature beats	9	2	1	0	12 (46)
Ventricular tachycardia	5	0	1	0	6 (23)
Complete heart block	4	1	0	1	6 (23)
Syncope	3	0	0	0	3 (12)
Left bundle branch block	0	1	0	0	1 (12)
Right bundle branch block	1	1	0	0	2
Congestive heart failure	2	6	0	0	8 (31)
Diagnosis of sarcoid in life	5	0	2	1	8 (31)
Corticosteroid therapy	2	0	0	1	3 (12)
Heart weight (g)					
Range	300–550	300–660	350, 570	310	300–660
Average	430	536	460	310	428
Cardiac granulomas					
Left ventricle	17	6	2	0	25 (96)
Ventricular septum	15	4	0	0	19 (73)
Right ventricle	10	2	0	0	12 (46)
Papillary muscle	11	5	1	0	17 (65)
Atria	2	1	0	0	3 (12)
None	0	0	0	1	1 (4)
Ventricular aneurysm	2	0	0	0	2 (8)
Cardiac mural thrombi	0	0	0	1	1 (4)
Noncardiac granulomas					
Lymph node	17	6	2	1	26 (100)
Lung	15	4	1	0	20 (77)
Liver	11	4	2	1	18 (69)
Spleen	11	4	2	1	18 (69)
Other	6	2	2	1	11 (42)

NOTE: Figures in parentheses are per cents.

* This average includes six patients whose initial manifestation of sarcoidosis was sudden death.

present at necropsy in the most cephalad portion of the muscular ventricular septum. In addition to the six patients with complete heart block, three others had **complete bundle branch block** (right in two; left in one); one of these patients also had episodes of ventricular tachycardia, and another had atrial fibrillation.

It is presumed that an arrhythmia or a conduction disturbance was the cause of **sudden death,** which was the mode of death in 17 (65 per cent) of the 26 patients. Sudden death was the initial manifestation of sarcoidosis in six (35 per cent) of the 17 patients who died suddenly, and in each, death occurred during exertion. In none of these six patients was an electrocardiogram ever recorded. Of the remaining 11 patients who died suddenly, five had recurring episodes of ventricular tachycardia, and four others had complete heart block, three of whom had episodes of syncope (Stokes-Adams attacks). Of the remaining two patients who died suddenly, one was known to have ventricular premature beats, but he had always been asymptomatic and without any recognized features of sarcoidosis; the second patient, a 26 year old woman, began to lose weight about three years before her death, had a persistent cough, a right Horner's syndrome, and pulmonary lesions and hilar lymphadenopathy. Fatal rapid atrial fibrillation developed shortly after the patient underwent an open biopsy of lung.

Congestive cardiac failure occurred in eight of the

TABLE III Cardiac Sarcoidosis Not Causing Cardiac Dysfunction: Clinical and Morphologic Observations in Nine Personally Studied Patients (Group IB) and in 15 Previously Described Patients (Group IIB)

Data	Group IB (9 patients)			Group IIB (15 patients)			Totals
	Respiratory Failure	Nonsarcoid Cardiac Dysfunction	Noncardiac and Nonpulmonary	Respiratory Failure	Nonsarcoid Cardiac Dysfunction	Noncardiac and Nonpulmonary	
Patients	4	3	2	10	3	2	24*
References	. . .	. . .	. . .	[51–59, 61]	[22, 63, 64]	[60, 62]	[22, 51–64]
Ages (yr)							
Range	30–59	28–50	38–43	28–58	40–68	72, 83	28–83
Average	40	39	40	45	52	77	45
Race							
Black	3	2	1	3	0	0	9 (37)
White	1	1	1	4	2	1	10 (42)
Unknown	0	0	0	3	1	1	5 (21)
Sex							
Male	2	2	0	8	2	2	16 (67)
Female	2	1	2	2	1	0	8 (33)
Duration of symptoms (mo)							
Range	24–96	10–168	0–12	5–84	36–54	. . .	0–96
Average	72	71	6	36	45		46
Atrial arrhythmia	0	0	0	1	0	0	1 (4)
Ventricular premature beats	0	0	0	0	1	0	1 (4)
Bundle branch block	0	0	0	0	1	1	2 (8)
Congestive heart failure	. . .	3	0	. . .	3	0	6 (25)
Diagnosis of sarcoid during life	4	1	0	8	2	0	10 (42)
Corticosteroid therapy	2	0	0	0	1	0	3 (12)
Heart weight (g)							
Range	300–400	370–950	280–460	250–420	520–870	340	250–950
Average	345	623	370	336	670	340	440
Cardiac granulomas							
Left ventricle	4	3	2	3/3	. . .	2	14/14 (100)
Ventricular septum	1	1	0	2/3	. . .	1	5/14 (36)
Right ventricle	2	2	1	3/3	. . .	2	10/14 (71)
Papillary muscle	. . .	1	. . .	0/3	. . .	. . .	1/6 (17)
Atria	0	0	0	0/3	. . .	. . .	0
Noncardiac granulomas							
Lymph node	4	3	2	9/9	3	2	23/23 (100)
Lung	4	2	2	9/9	1	2	20/23 (87)
Liver	4	3	2	6/9	1	2	18/23 (78)
Spleen	4	2	2	7/9	1	2	18/23 (78)
Other	3	2	1	5/9	1	0	12/23 (52)

NOTE: Figures in parentheses are per cents.

* None of these 24 patients had ventricular tachycardia, complete heart block, syncope, cardiac aneurysm, intracardiac thrombi, or completely healed myocardial granulomas.

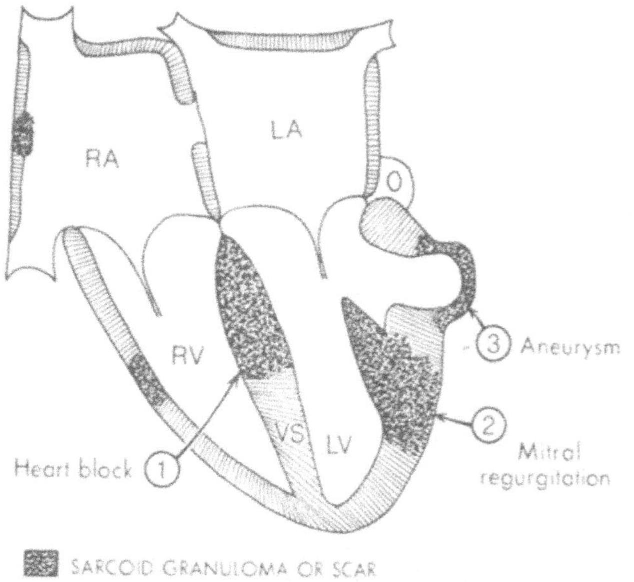

Figure 1. *Diagram showing the most common sites of sarcoid granulomas or scars in the heart and the most frequent functional consequences of these lesions.*

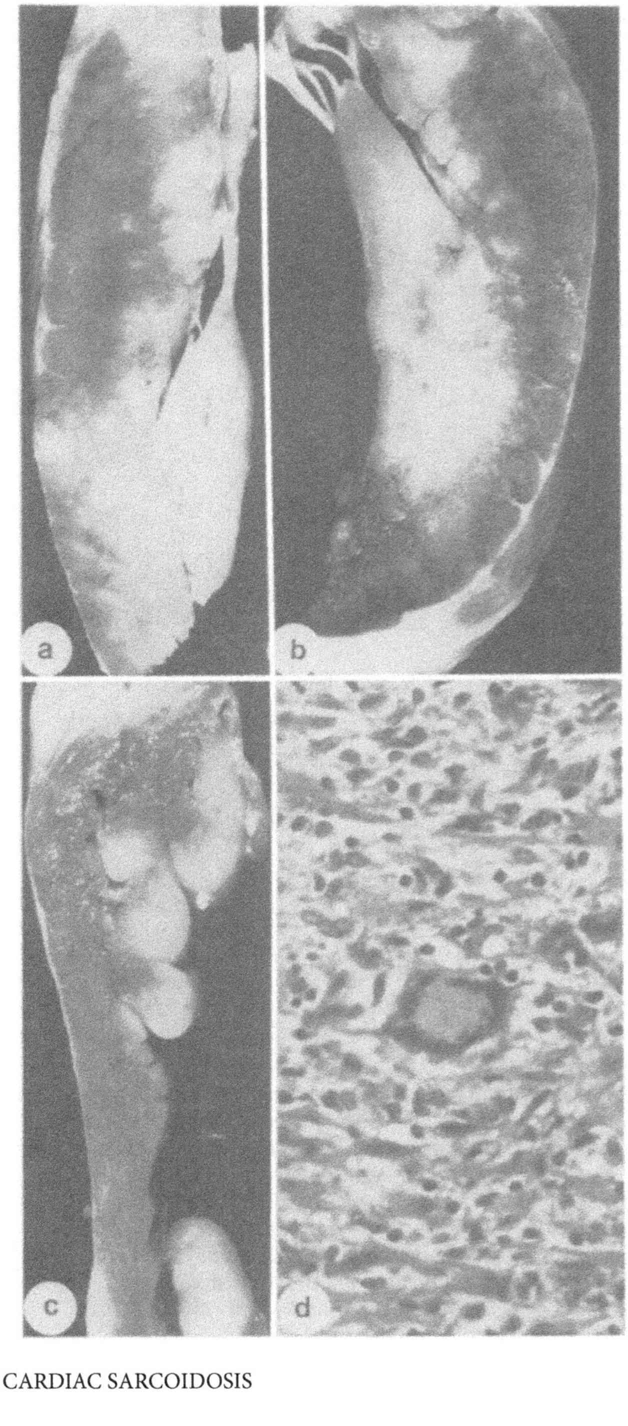

Figure 2. *The heart in a 26 year old black woman (A-70-541) who had been asymptomatic until 10 days before her death when dyspnea appeared. The dyspnea rapidly worsened, and when the patient was hospitalized on the day of death, she was in acute pulmonary edema. The blood pressure was 80/70 mm Hg, heart rate 160 beats/min and a grade 3-4/6 pansystolic blowing murmur, which radiated to the axilla, was audible. A chest roentgenogram showed congested lungs, cardiomegaly and prominent hilar adenopathy. Electrocardiogram showed nonspecific S-T segment and T-wave changes and atrial hypertrophy. Complete heart block developed and the patient died shortly thereafter.* ***a*** *and* ***b,*** *longitudinal sections of left ventricular free wall at sites of the papillary muscles. The latter are totally replaced by firm, white deposits, several of which also infiltrate the free wall.* ***c,*** *longitudinal section of right atrial wall showing similar white deposits.* ***d,*** *histologic section of a portion of a white deposit in the heart showing typical sarcoid granulomas. Similar hard granulomas were present in lymph nodes, liver, spleen and lung. Hematoxylin and eosin stain; original magnification × 400 (**d**), reduced by 12 per cent.*

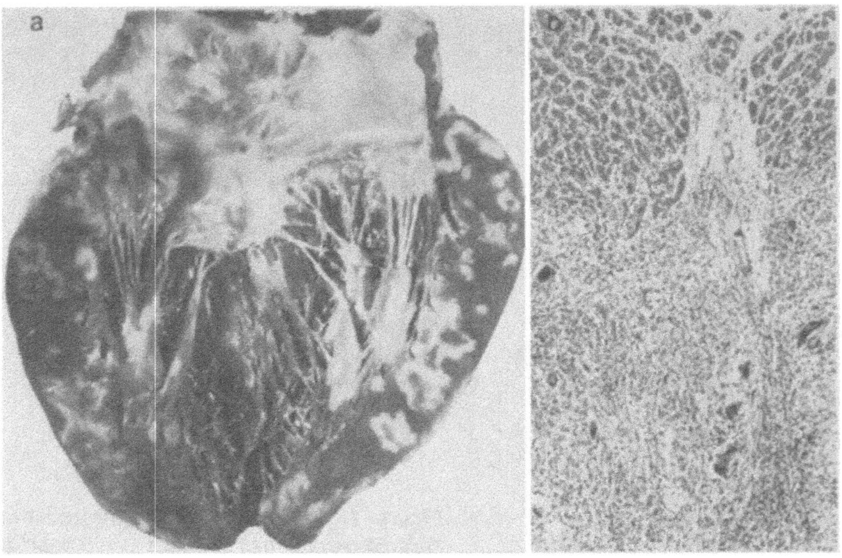

Figure 3. *Opened left atrium, mitral valve and left ventricle (**a**) and photomicrograph of a portion of the left ventricular wall (**b**) in a 28 year old black man (A-70-55) who died suddenly on his job as a construction worker. He had been well until two days earlier when he complained of "pain in his neck," but this had not prevented him from performing his usual activities. He had never sought medical care. At necropsy, sarcoid granulomas were found in the mediastinal lymph nodes, lung and heart. The heart weighed 420 g. Numerous sarcoid granulomas are present in the left ventricular free wall and in both papillary muscles. The posteromedial one is virtually replaced by the granulomas. Hematoxylin and eosin stain (**b**); original magnification × 100, reduced by 26 per cent.*

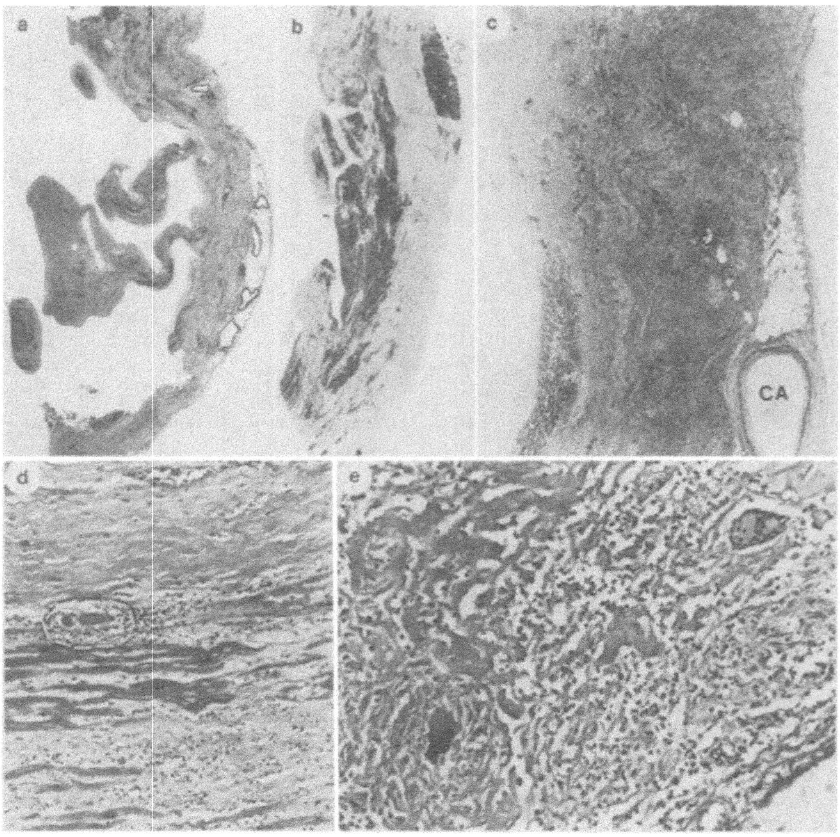

Figure 4. *Photomicrographs of the posterior left ventricular free wall in a 44 year old, extremely obese (260 pounds), white woman (A73-128) in whom evidence of congestive cardiac failure developed months before her death. A chest roentgenogram showed mild cardiomegaly and "pulmonary congestion." Several days before death, ventricular tachycardia developed suddenly. Episodes of this arrhythmia occurred until her death. Diagnosis of sarcoid was not suspected during life. **a, b, c,** longitudinal sections of left ventricular posterior wall at three different sites. In **a** and **c** there is complete transmural replacement of the wall primarily by fibrous tissue which contains occasional granuloma. The posteromedial papillary muscle is also completely replaced by sarcoid (**a**). Mainly the epicardial half of the portion shown in **b** is replaced. The coronary arteries (CA), one of which is shown in **c,** were wide open. In **d** only one granuloma (dashed circle) is present but the amount of fibrous tissue is extensive. In **e** more granulomas are seen. Far more granulomas were present in the lymph nodes than in the heart. Some also were found in the liver, spleen and lungs. Masson trichrome stain (**a** and **b**), hematoxylin and eosin stain (**c**, **d** and **e**); original magnification × 3 (**a** and **b**), × 15 (**c**), × 140 (**d**) and × 200 (**e**), reduced by 40 per cent.*

26 patients. Two of the eight patients had mild failure and died suddenly; the other six had progressive and eventually fatal failure. The left ventricular walls were extensively infiltrated by sarcoid granulomas in all eight patients with congestive cardiac failure. Of the six patients with severe, fatal heart failure, two had loud (grade 3–4/6) precordial, apical, systolic murmurs consistent with mitral regurgitation. At necropsy, both patients had extensive infiltration of their left ventricular papillary muscles by sarcoid granulomas; thus each had papillary muscle dysfunction as a result of myocardial sarcoidosis. Two patients had changes on the electrocardiogram that suggested recent myocardial infarction; one patient presented with acute failure, was symptomatic for only about one month and, during life, was considered to have the failure on the basis of acute myocardial infarction. Two patients, each of whom had had chronic failure for at least six months, had an acute exacerbation of the failure several days before death; at necropsy, each had large pulmonary emboli.

Recurring pericardial effusion was the cause of cardiac dysfunction in two of the 26 patients. The

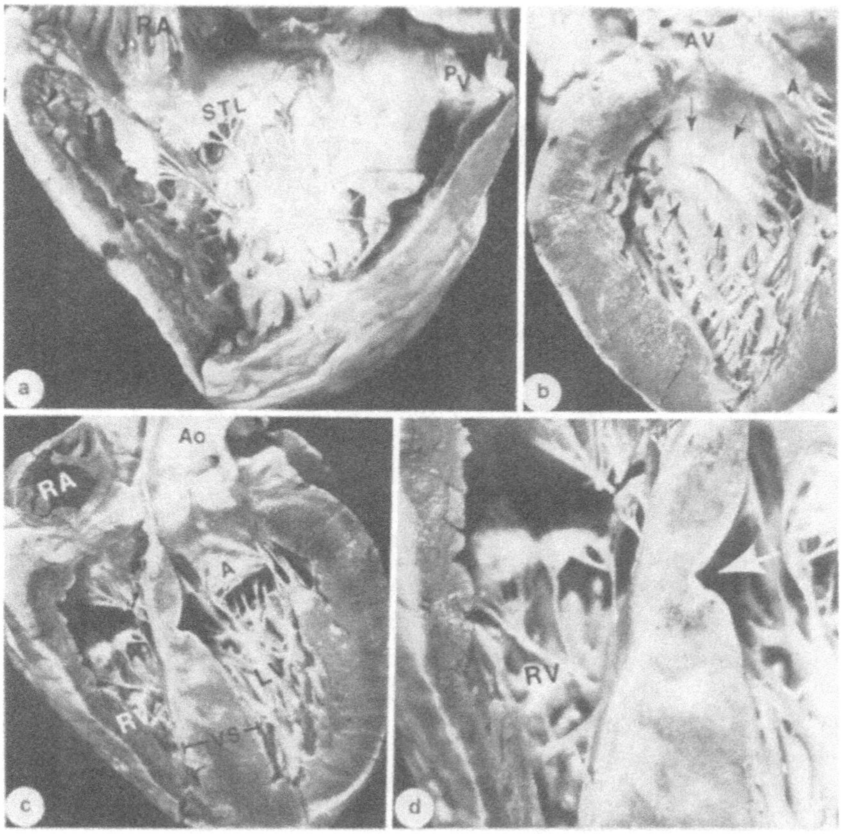

Figure 5. *Heart in a 30 year old black man (73-12-1146) who, three years before his death, was found to have bilateral pulmonary infiltrates. Open biopsy at that time disclosed sarcoidosis. He was asymptomatic until about 12 months before death when he noted occasional palpitations. Seven months before death he had the sudden onset of dyspnea, severe weakness and sweating, and he was found to have supraventricular tachycardia with a ventricular rate of 260 beats/min. Cardioversion restored his rhythm to sinus mechanism. An electrocardiogram shortly thereafter showed complete right bundle branch block, left ventricular hypertrophy and changes suggesting anteroseptal myocardial infarction of indeterminate age. A chest roentgenogram showed bilateral pulmonary infiltrates. Other electrocardiograms during this hospitalization showed atrial, nodal and ventricular premature beats, and periodic nodal tachycardia. Prednisone therapy was started at this time, initially 40 mg daily, and three months before death, 25 mg daily. The supraventricular tachycardia recurred thereafter about once a month until death despite prednisone, procainamide, diphenylhydantoin, and transiently, transvenous pacemaker, therapy. He was found dead in a hotel room while on a trip. At necropsy, the heart weighed 450 g. A small focus of fibrous pericardial adhesions was present posteriorly. The walls of both cardiac ventricles were hypertrophied. The endocardium of the right ventricular aspect of the ventricular septum was white and thick (**a**). RA = right atrium; PV = pulmonic valve; STL = septal tricuspid leaflet. A small indentation surrounded by white thick endocardium (**arrows**) was present on the left ventricular aspect of the ventricular septum (**b**). On longitudinal section (**c**) the cephalad portion of the ventricular septum (VS) was thinned and extensively infiltrated by firm white tissue which histologically was typical of sarcoid. LV = left ventricle; RV = right ventricle; A = anterior mitral leaflet; Ao = aorta. A close-up view of the sarcoid-infiltrated ventricular septum is shown in **d.** The indentation (**arrow**) of the ventricular septum is well shown.*

effusions had recurred over periods of 16 and 18 months, respectively, and both patients had huge cardiac silhouettes on chest roentgenogram. The diagnosis of sarcoidosis was established in each by biopsy of parietal pericardium one and two days, respectively, before death. At open biopsy, each patient had approximately 800 ml of serous pericardial effusion; at necropsy, each had sarcoid granulomas in the parietal pericardium, and both had left ventricular myocardial granulomas. Granulomas in one patient were small and in the second patient, huge.

Morphologic Observations. The weight of the heart in the 26 patients ranged from 310 to 700 g (average 461 g). The average weight among the 17 patients who died suddenly was less than that in the six patients with fatal congestive cardiac failure. Cardiac granulomas were observed grossly in 25 of the 26 hearts, and in the remaining one transmural myocardial scars were present. Sarcoid granulomas were present in the left ventricular free wall of all 25 patients, in the ventricular septum in at least 19 patients, in the right ventricular wall in 12 patients, in the right atrial wall in three patients and in the left atrial wall in two. The granulomas were most extensive in the left ventricular free wall and usually transmural (involving more than half of the thickness of the wall) (Figures 1 through 4). The deposits in the atrial wall were small (<1 cm) in all but one patient (Figure 2), in whom they were extensive in the right

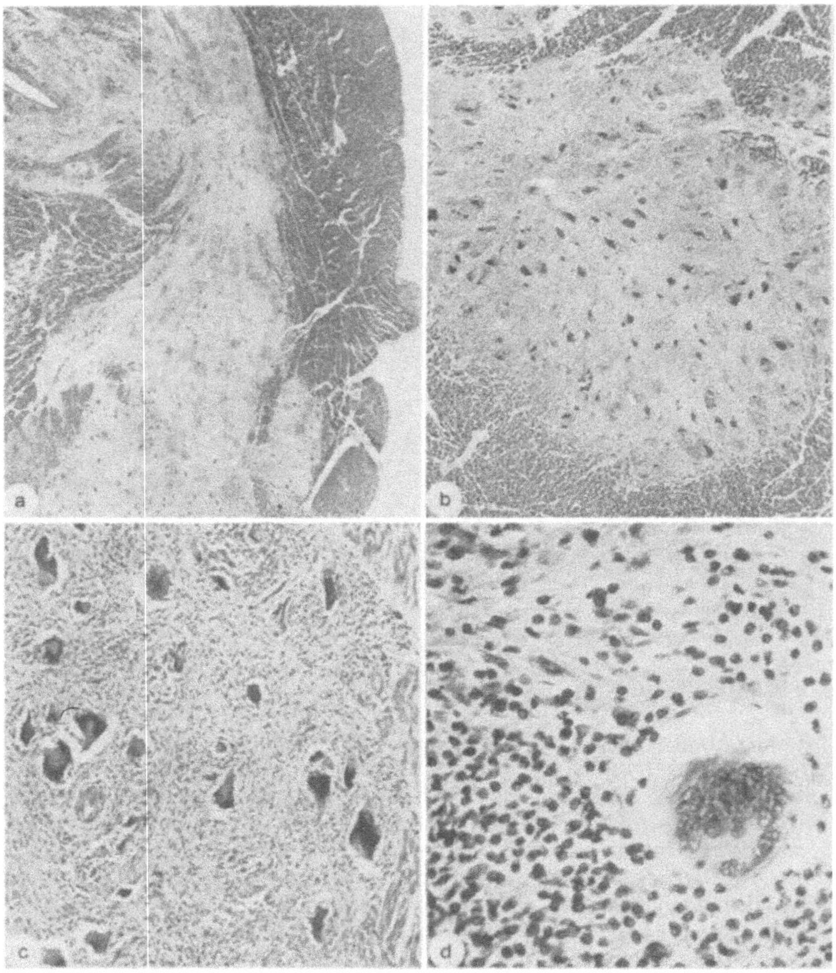

Figure 6. *Extensive, myocardial sarcoid in a 49 year old extremely obese (220 pounds) Indian woman (A-5559) who had been asymptomatic until two months before death when she fainted, and an electrocardiogram showed complete heart block with a ventricular rate of 32 beats/min. A chest roentgenogram disclosed mild cardiomegaly. Thereafter, she became quite dyspneic with only mild exertion. She collapsed while in the bathroom, and resuscitation was unsuccessful. Diagnosis of sarcoidosis was never suspected during life. At necropsy, the heart weighed 430 g. The entire cephalad portion of the ventricular septum, the entire anterolateral papillary muscle and several portions of left ventricular free wall were replaced by sarcoid granulomas.* ***a,*** *low power view of the ventricular septum showing extensive replacement of myocardium by sarcoid.* ***b, c*** *and* ***d,*** *progressive higher power views showing numerous giant cells, mononuclear cells and fibrous tissue. Hematoxylin and eosin stains; original magnification* $\times$ *11 (**a**),* $\times$ *35 (**b**),* $\times$ *130 (**c**) and* $\times$ *185 (**d**), reduced by 40 per cent.*

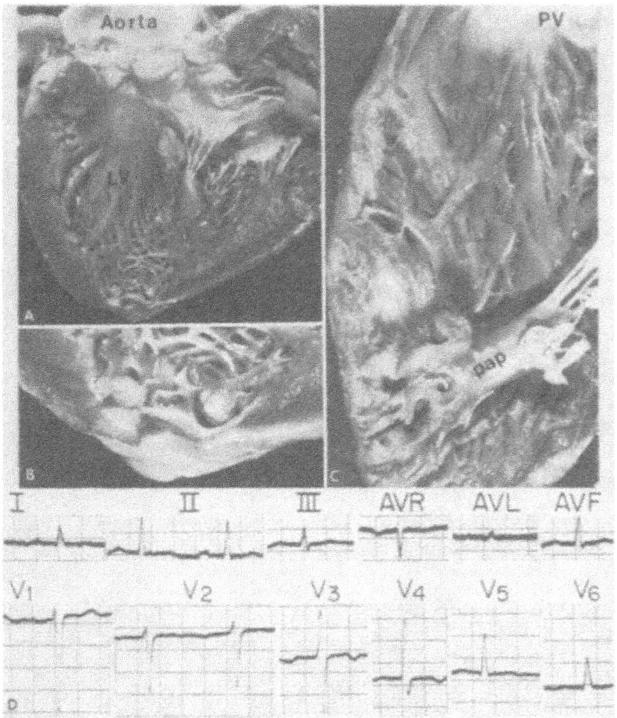

Figure 7. *Heart and electrocardiogram in a 34 year old man (A68-10) who noted swelling in his neck at age 29. Biopsy of the excised lump at age 30 disclosed that it consisted of lymph nodes infiltrated by hard granulomas. A diagnosis of sarcoidosis therefore was made. The liver was within normal limits on biopsy at age 31. A chest roentgenogram showed prominent bilateral hilar adenopathy, and prednisone therapy (10 to 20 mg daily) was begun and continued thereafter until his death. Five months later cryptococcal meningitis developed, but it was eradicated by amphotericin therapy. One year before death marked hypercalcemia developed. About one month before death a high degree of atrioventricular block developed, which at times progressed to complete heart block. The patient died of complications of peptic ulcer perforation. At necropsy the heart weighed 320 g. Both ventricular cavities were mildly dilated. Mural thrombi were present at the apices of both ventricles. The apical left ventricular wall beneath the thrombi was fibrotic; a small area of scarring was present in the basal anterior left ventricular wall, and the anterior right ventricular wall was focally scarred. Histologic study of the scarred areas disclosed some mononuclear cells but no giant cells. The area of the atrioventricular node and bundle was serially sectioned: considerable scarring with some mononuclear cells was present in the conduction tissue, but the node and bundle and proximal bundle branches were not interrupted at any point. Although no granulomas were observed in this patient's heart, it is nevertheless highly likely that the myocardial scars were the result of "healed" sarcoid granulomas. The myocardial scarring, for example, was similar to that observed in the lymph nodes, and the coronary arteries were normal. The healing appears to have been the result of steroid therapy given for three years.* ***A,*** *opened left ventricle (LV). At the apex is a thrombus, better seen in* ***B.*** *The myocardium beneath the thrombus is scarred.* ***C,*** *right ventricular wall shows severe focal scarring. Pap = papillary muscle.* ***D,*** *electrocardiograms recorded three days before death.*

atrium. The granulomas grossly were white and firm. In addition to the left ventricular free wall, granulomas often were observed in the left ventricular papillary muscles (at least 17 patients) (Figures 1, 2 and 3) and in the ventricular septum (at least 19 patients), primarily its cephalad portion (Figures 5 and 6). Of the six patients with complete heart block, five had granulomas in the most cephalad portion of the muscular ventricular septum (Figures 5 and 6), and one had scar tissue in this area (Figure 7). In the one patient in whom serial sections were studied (Figure 5), the atrioventricular bundle and the proximal portions of the right and left bundle branches were partially destroyed by granulomas. In a number of patients, large portions of the left ventricular free wall and ventricular septum were completely replaced by sarcoid granulomas (Figures 2 through 6). The white granulomas usually were visible on the endocardial surface of the left ventricle and, in several patients, they were grossly visible on the epicardial surface. Electron microscopic examination of a sarcoid granuloma in the myocardium was performed in one patient; ultrastructurally, the granulomas were similar to those present in the lungs (Figure 8). In several patients without grossly visible epicardial granulomas, histologic examination of the atrioventricular sulci and epicardium disclosed sarcoid granulomas. In each of the two patients with recurring pericardial effusions, sarcoid granulomas were present in both visceral and parietal pericardia (Figure 9).

Left ventricular aneurysm was present at necropsy in two patients, each of whom had myocardial granulomas. Sudden death was the initial manifestation of sarcoidosis in both patients.

In addition to occurring in the lymph nodes, granulomas consistent with sarcoidosis were present in the lung in 20 patients; in the liver in 18; in the spleen in 18 and in other organs or tissues in 11. The average weight of the liver and spleen was only slightly increased despite the presence of granulomas in these organs. The liver ranged in weight from 1,250 to 2,300 g (average 1,755 g) and the spleen, from 120 to 350 g (average 244 g). The weights of the lungs (together) were usually increased: they ranged from 800 to 1,600 g (average 1,132 g).

Observations in the Patients in Whom Cardiac Dysfunction, if Present, was Not Secondary to Cardiac Sarcoidosis (Group IB). In contrast to the 26 patients described, each of these nine patients had small (microscopic-sized in eight) myocardial sarcoid granulomas (Table III). Four had extensive pulmonary sarcoidosis resulting in cor pulmonale. Three had cardiac dysfunction on the basis of nonsarcoid cardiac conditions: valvular heart disease in two causing pure aortic regurgitation of uncertain etiology in one, and combined mitral and aortic regurgitation in one, presumably rheumatic in origin (this patient underwent mitral valve replacement three months before a fatal cerebral embolus); the third patient, a 50 year old man, had severe coronary atherosclerosis with a documented acute myocardial infarction nine years before his death and congestive cardiac failure probably on that basis. The myocardial granulomas in each of these three patients were minute and visible only by histologic examination. None of these nine patients had arrhythmias or conduction disturbances. None of the five patients without respiratory insufficiency had symptoms or signs definitely attributable to sarcoidosis. The diagnosis of

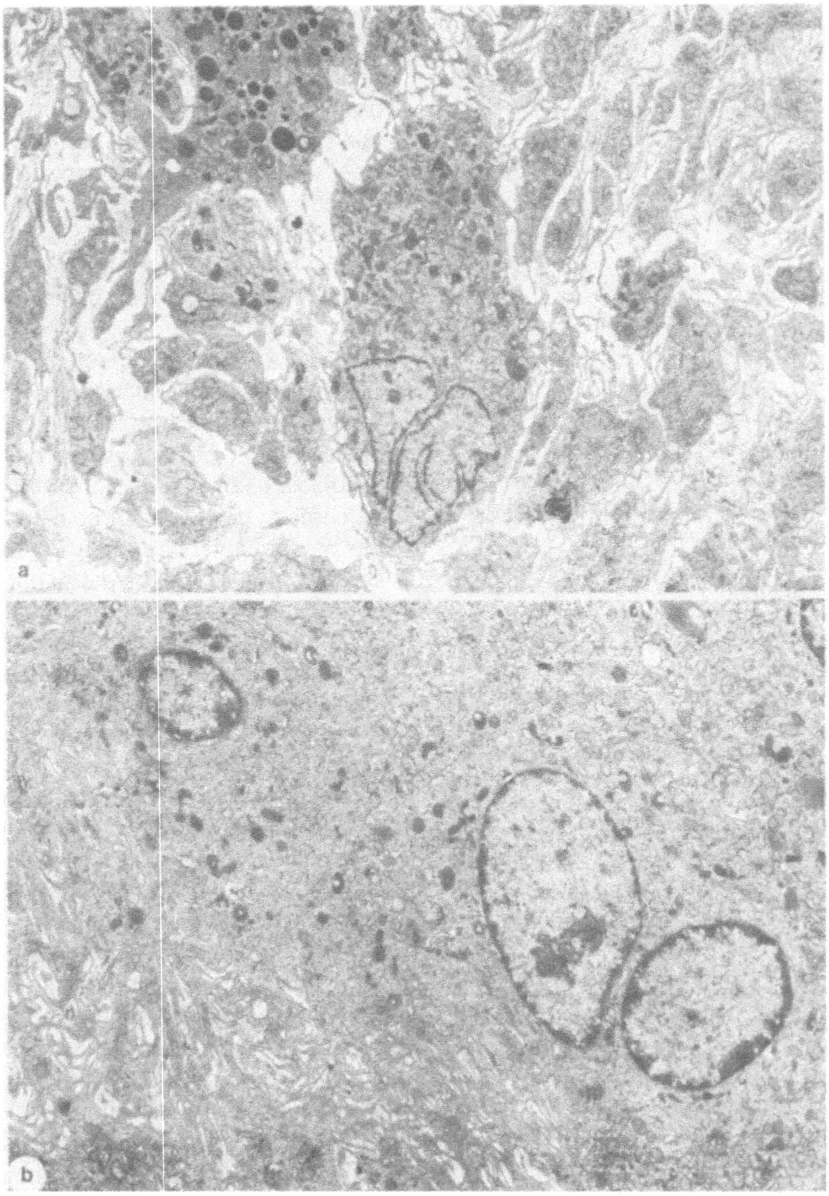

Figure 8. *Electron micrographs of portions of sarcoid granuloma from a biopsy specimen of lung tissue from a 24 year old white man. Similar granulomas were observed ultrastructurally in the myocardium in the one patient examined in the present study, but preservation of the myocardial tissue was not nearly as good as that of the lung biopsy specimen.* ***a,*** *in this electron micrograph an epithelioid cell is present in the central area; it has a multilobulated nucleus and numerous cytoplasmic dense bodies. The surface of this cell is highly irregular, with many flap- and pocket-like projections. Similar projections are present on the surfaces of adjacent cells. A macrophage-like cell is present at the upper left; it contains many large dense bodies.* ***b,*** *portion of multinucleated giant cell (same tissue as in* ***a****) showing parts of 4 nuclei and moderate numbers of dense bodies, mitochondria and cisterns of endoplasmic reticulum. The surface of this cell (lower left) is highly convoluted with complex, interdigitating folds. Original magnification × 6,000 (****a****) and × 7,500 (****b****), reduced by 38 per cent.*

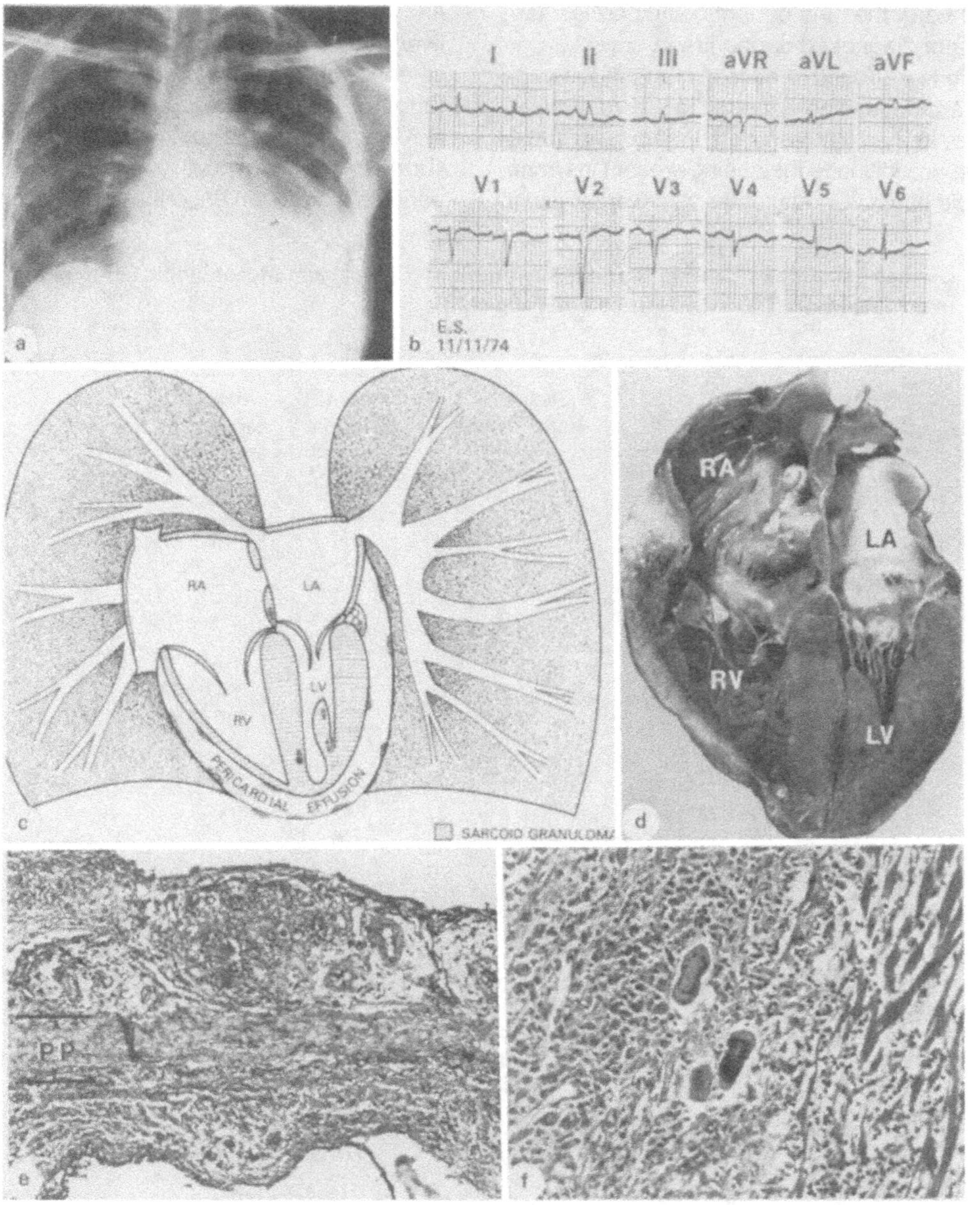

Figure 9. *Chest roentgenogram, electrocardiogram, diagram of heart and lungs, longitudinal cut of heart, and photomicrographs of parietal pericardium and left ventricular papillary muscle in a 47 year old black woman (74-A-223) who was well until 15 months before death when she noted exertional dyspnea, cough and retrosternal chest pain. Hospitalization a month later disclosed distended neck veins, a pericardial friction rub and bilateral pulmonary rales. A chest roentgenogram showed pulmonary "congestion" and mild cardiomegaly. A right-sided cardiac angiogram disclosed a large pericardial effusion. During her four month period in the hospital, infiltrates appeared in the lower lobes of both lungs, but a definite diagnosis was not made. During the next 10 months, she had only dyspnea on severe exertion and an occasional nonproductive cough. A week before death, she had the sudden appearance of severe dyspnea. Physical examination disclosed pulsus paradoxicus (12 mm Hg), distended neck veins and hepatosplenomegaly; roentgenography (**a**) disclosed bilateral pleural effusions, a large cardiac silhouette and interstitial pulmonary infiltrates. An electrocardiogram (**b**) showed low voltage and sinus tachycardia. An echocardiogram showed an echo-free space behind the posterior left ventricular wall. The pulmonary arterial pressure was 30/10 (mean 15) mm Hg. At open thoracotomy (for diagnostic purposes), 800 ml of straw-colored fluid was found in the pericardial sac (protein content = 2.5 g/100 ml; glucose = 105 mg/100 ml). The patient died three days later from progressive "respiratory insufficiency." At necropsy, many sarcoid granulomas were found in both lungs (**c**), hilar lymph nodes, liver and spleen. The parietal pericardium was thickened and contained many sarcoid granulomas (**e**). No lesions were noted on gross examination of the myocardium (**d**), but histologic study did disclose several sarcoid granulomas in the left ventricular free wall and papillary muscles. Granulomas also were present in the epicardium (**c**). The thickness of the normal parietal pericardium (PP) is shown in (**e**). Hematoxylin and eosin stains; original magnification × 85 (**e**) and × 220 (**f**), reduced by 38 per cent.*

noncardiac sarcoidosis was established by biopsy during life in five of the nine patients, and cardiac sarcoidosis was not diagnosed during life in any.

Granulomas were found at necropsy in the left ventricular myocardium in nine patients, in the ventricular septum in two, in the right ventricle in five, and in the atrium in none. In addition to their being present in lymph nodes in all nine patients, granulomas also were present in the lungs in eight, the liver in nine, the spleen in eight and in other organs or tissues in six. The weights of the liver ranged from 830 to 2,600 g (average 1,907 g); the spleen, from 70 to 400 g (average 211 g); and the lungs together, from 760 to 2,800 g (average 1,336 g).

Review of Data on Previously Described Patients with Cardiac Sarcoidosis (Group II). At least 78 necropsy patients have been described with sarcoid granulomas

TABLE IV Cardiac Sarcoidosis Causing Cardiac Dysfunction: Clinical and Morphologic Observations in 63 Previously Described Patients (Group IIA)

Data	Mode of Death					Totals
	Sudden	Congestive Heart Failure	Pericardial Effusion	Non-cardiac	Uncertain	
Patients (no.)	43	14	1	1	4	63
References	[1–34]	[10, 33, 35–44]	[47]	[2]	[48–54]	[1–51]
Age (yr)						
Range	18–76	24–67	27	42	18–38	18–76
Average	43	33	27	42	27	40
Race						
Black	13	10	1	1	2	27 (43)
White	14	2	0	0	1	17 (27)
Unknown or other	16	2	0	0	1	19 (30)
Sex						
Male	18*	9	0	1	2	30/62 (48)
Female	24*	5	1	0	2	32/62 (52)
Duration of symptoms (mo)						
Range	0–180	25–72	60	108	2–12	0–180
Average	27†	29§	60	108	7	28
Atrial arrhythmia	5	4	0	...	2	11 (17)
Ventricular premature beats	12	5	1	...	3	21 (33)
Ventricular tachycardia	8	4	0	...	1	13 (21)
Complete heart block	16	0	0	1	2	19 (30)
Syncope	14	1	0	1	1	17 (27)
Left bundle branch block	2	1	0	...	1	4 }
Right bundle branch block	8	2	0	...	1	11 } (32)
Indeterminate bundle block	3	1	0	...	1	5 }
Congestive heart failure	10	14	1	...	2	27 (43)
Diagnosis of sarcoid in life	10	5	0	...	1	16 (25)
Corticosteroid therapy	8	3	0	0	1	12 (19)
Heart weight (g)						
Range	225–640	320–660	745	...	300–450	225–745
Average	439‡	549§	745	...	385¶	476
Cardiac granulomas						
Left ventricle	28/30	9/9	1	0	2/2	40/41 (98)
Ventricular septum	27/30	4/9	1	0	1/2	33/41 (80)
Right ventricle	10/30	5/9	1	0	0/2	16/41 (39)
Papillary muscle	10/30	2/9	...	0	0/2	12/41 (29)
Atria	9/30	2/9	1	0	0/2	12/41 (29)
None	2	1	0	1	0	4 (6)
Ventricular aneurysm	4	2	0	0	0	6 (15)
Cardiac mural thrombi	0	4	0	0	0	4 (10)
Noncardiac granulomas						
Lymph node	41/41	12/12	1	1	4	59/59 (100)
Lung	35/41	9/12	1	0	4	49/59 (83)
Liver	22/41	8/12	1	0	4	35/59 (59)
Spleen	20/41	7/12	0	0	3	30/59 (51)
Other	9/41	6/12	1	0	1	17/59 (29)

* Sex not stated in one patient.

† Information from 30 patients; average includes four patients whose initial manifestation of sarcoidosis was sudden death. The average in the 26 patients with symptoms was 32 months.

‡ Eighteen patients.

§ Ten patients.

¶ Two patients.

(75 patients) or nonischemic myocardial scars, i.e., healed granulomas (three patients), in their hearts and sarcoid granulomas in at least one other body organ (Tables III and IV). The 78 patients were subdivided into two groups: (1) 63 patients with cardiac dysfunction resulting from extensive cardiac sarcoidosis (group IIA) [1–51] (Table IV) and (2) 15 patients with minute cardiac granulomas and either no (12 patients) cardiac dysfunction [51–62] or cardiac dysfunction (three patients) [22,63,64] not on the basis of cardiac sarcoidosis (group IIB) (Table III). Observations in these two groups of previously described cases are added to those in the personally studied patients and summarized in Table V.

Analysis of these 63 patients (group IIA, Table III) indicates that 43 died suddenly [1–34], 14 from progressive congestive cardiac failure [10,33,35–46], one from recurring pericardial effusion [47], one from noncardiac (suicide) [2] and four from unknown causes [48–51]. Sudden death was the initial manifestation of sarcoidosis in four of the 43 patients who died suddenly [4,6,12,27]; in the other 39 patients, symptoms were present from five days to 180 months (average 27 months). Electrocardiograms, obtained in 53 of the 63 patients, disclosed atrial **arrhythmias** in 11 [5,25–27,31,33,36,42,46,48,51], **ventricular premature beats** in 19 [7,12,16–18,20,27,28,31,34,35,37,40,45,46,49–51], **ventricular tachycardia** in 12 [10,17,27–29,32–35,37,39,40], **complete heart block** in 19 [2,7,11,13–16,20–24,30,31,49,50], second degree heart block in four [14,24,25,47], prolonged (>0.20 sec) P-R interval in five [18,27,36,40,46] and **complete bundle branch block** in 18 (left = three, right = 11, indeterminate = four) [5,7,11,14,16,18–20,25,26,31,33,36,41,46,51]. None of the 19 patients with complete heart block had ventricular tachycardia. Clinical evidence of **congestive cardiac failure** was present in 26 (50 per cent) [7,10,17,19,23,25–27,29,32,33,35–46,48,51] of the 52 patients in whom it was mentioned. The diagnosis of sarcoidosis was established during life in only 16 (25 per cent) of the 63 patients [3,10,14–16,22,27,29,31,34,37,38,40,44,46,51]. Twelve of the 63 patients received corticosteroid therapy at some time [15,19,20,22,27–29,34,44–46,51].

At necropsy, the **cardiac weight,** available in 31 of the 63 patients, ranged from 225 to 745 g (average 476 g). Although granulomas were present in "the heart" or "myocardium" of 60 patients, the **specific chambers involved** were mentioned in 44 patients: the left ventricle in 40 (91 per cent), the ventricular septum in 33 (75 per cent), the right ventricle in 16 (36 per cent) and

TABLE V Cardiac Sarcoidosis: Summary of Personally Studied and Previously Described Patients

Data	Causing Cardiac Dysfunction (Groups IA and IIA)	Not Causing Cardiac Dysfunction (Groups 1B and IIB)
Patients (no.)	89	24
Age (yr)		
Range	18–76	28–83
Average	40	45
Race		
Black	41	9
White	27	10
Unknown	0	3
Sex		
Male	45	16
Female	44	5
Unknown	0	3
Symptoms (mo)		
Range	0–180	0–96
Average	22	46
Syncope	20 (22)	0
Congestive heart failure	35 (39)	6 (25)
Atrial arrhythmia	15 (17)	1 (4)
Ventricular premature beats	33 (37)	1 (4)
Ventricular tachycardia	19 (21)	0
Complete heart block	25 (28)	0
Complete bundle branch block	23 (26)	2 (8)
Diagnosis of sarcoid in life	24 (27)	15 (62)
Corticosteroid treatment	15 (17)	3 (12)
Ventricular aneurysm	8 (9)	0
Intracardiac thrombi	5 (6)	0

NOTE: Figures in parentheses are per cents.

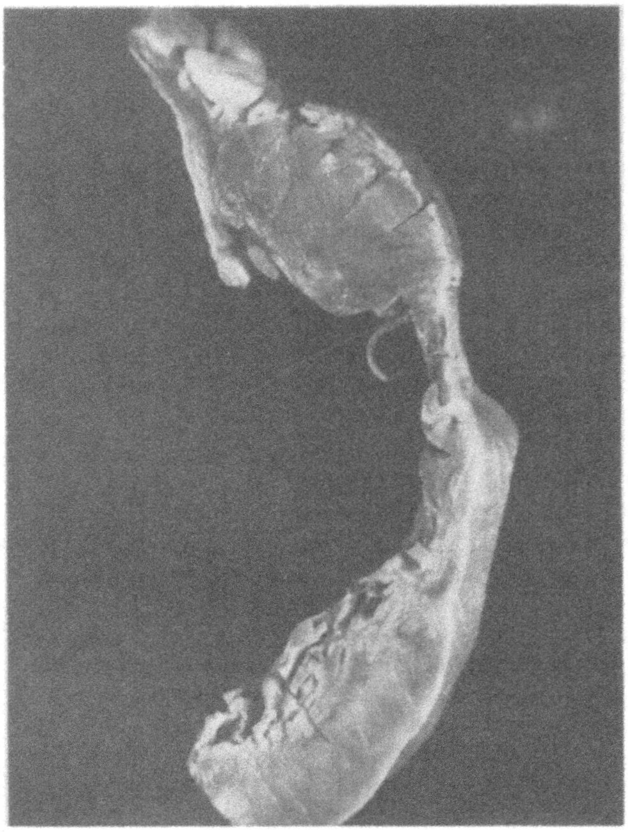

Figure 10. *Longitudinal section of left ventricular free wall showing an area of thinning which during life resulted in an aneurysm. This 49 year old black woman (A72-144), reported earlier by Chun and associates [34] and also examined by one of us (WCR), had 20 episodes of ventricular tachycardia during a 38-month period. She was treated with prednisone most of that time. She died suddenly. At necropsy, the wall of the left ventricular aneurysm consisted entirely of fibrous tissue and the coronary arteries were normal. No sarcoid granulomas were present in the heart but they were present in lymph nodes, spleen, liver and bone marrow. The heart weighed 470 g. It is believed that sarcoid granulomas were present in the heart at one time but that the prednisone therapy caused their healing with development of the above illustrated aneurysm.*

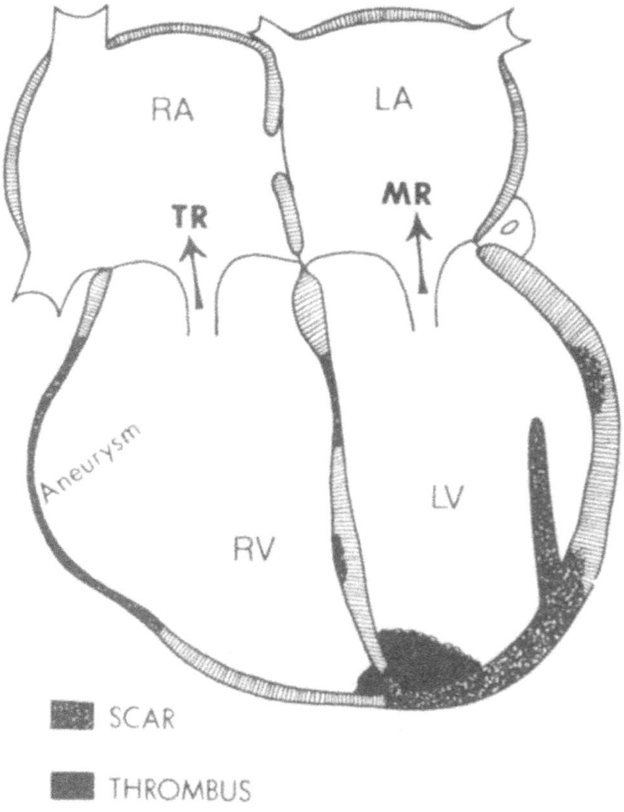

Figure 11. *Diagram of heart in a 37 year old white man (BIH A74-275) who was described in a New England Journal of Medicine CPC by Harthorne and Freiman [46]. (The heart was examined by one of us [WCR] through the courtesy of Walter H. Abelmann and David G. Freiman.) This case is of particular importance because the patient's course was eight years. During this period he had multiple arrhythmias, bilateral bundle branch block with prolongation of the P-R interval, systemic emboli, and progressive cardiomegaly, so that by necropsy both ventricles were enormously dilated and the right ventricular wall, so thinned that it was aneurysmal. Scars also were present in the left ventricular free wall and ventricular septum but no granulomas were present in the heart. Indeed, although sarcoid granulomas had been present in lymph nodes in an earlier biopsy, at necropsy no sarcoid granulomas were present in any organ. It is believed that corticosteroid therapy (two years) contributed to the disappearance of the granulomas. His heart at necropsy was very similar to the typical heart of idiopathic cardiomyopathy of the ventricular dilated type except for the presence of the healed granulomas (scars).*

the atrium in 12 (right atrium in eight, left atrium in seven and unspecified in one) (27 per cent). In at least 12 patients [1,3–6,10,12,14,18,32,40,43] sarcoid granulomas were stated to be present in one or more papillary muscles. The cardiac granulomas were visible grossly in all patients. One or more **ventricular aneurysms** were present in six patients [19,29,33,34,44,46] (Figures 10 and 11), and intracardiac thrombi in four patients [10,35,42,46] (Figure 11), all of whom had congestive cardiac failure. The specific location of sarcoid granulomas in organs other than the heart was described in 59 patients: lymph nodes in 59 (100 per cent); lung in 49 (83 per cent); liver in 35 (59 per cent); spleen in 31 (53 per cent) and other organs in 17 (29 per cent).

Observations in the previously described 15 patients in whom cardiac dysfunction, if present, was not secondary to cardiac sarcoidosis (group IIB) are summarized in Table II [22,51–64]. In contrast to the patients in group IIA, men were more numerous than women (12:3), the duration of symptoms was longer (average 38 months), arrhythmias and conduction defects were infrequent, the diagnosis of sarcoidosis was made in life in 10 of the 15 patients, and one patient died suddenly. The heart weights, available in 10 patients, were normal in seven and increased in the three patients with cardiac dysfunction from valvular disease of nonsarcoid origin. The cardiac sarcoid granulomas were minute in all 15 patients and usually visible only by histologic examination. Other body organs involved by sarcoid included the lymph nodes in all 15 patients, the lung in 12, the liver in nine, the spleen in 10 and other body organs or tissues in six.

COMMENTS

Study of our 35 patients (group I) and the 78 previously described necropsy patients (group II) allows certain general conclusions regarding cardiac sarcoidosis, and these items will be discussed in the following order: (1) the portions of the heart involved anatomically by sarcoid granulomas; (2) the determinants of whether or not cardiac sarcoidosis causes cardiac dysfunction; (3) the clinical types of cardiac dysfunction and their probable anatomic explanations; (4) the determinants of whether or not cardiac dysfunction from cardiac sarcoidosis is diagnosed clincally; (5) the modes of death and length of illness; (6) the effect of corticosteroid therapy on cardiac sarcoid granulomas and (7) the differences between cardiac sarcoidosis and idiopathic granulomatous (giant cell) myocarditis.

No portion of the heart is immune to infiltration by sarcoid granulomas. The granulomas may involve the pericardium, myocardium and endocardium, but of the three, the myocardium is, by far, the one most frequently involved. The portion of myocardium most frequently involved by sarcoid granulomas is the left ventricular free wall, followed by the ventricular septum, the right ventricle and, lastly, the atrial wall. Why the left ventricular free wall is the one most frequently involved and the atrial wall the one least frequently involved is uncertain, but the explanation may simply be that the largest fraction of the total myocardial mass is in the left ventricle, including the ventricular septum, and the smallest fraction is in the atrium. (Interestingly, the left ventricular wall also is the most frequent portion of myocardium invaded by secondary neoplasms of the heart [65–67].) Sarcoid granulomas within the left ventricle appear to be most common in the papillary muscles and in the free walls immediately beneath them. The cephalad half of the ventricular septum is more often involved than the caudal half. It is probable that the left ventricular papillary muscles and the cephalad portion of the ventricular septum are the preferential locations in the heart for sarcoid granulomas, but since these sites often are not incised at necropsy small granulomas in these locations may be missed. Thus, it is possible that the frequency of cardiac involvement by granulomas in patients with sarcoidosis may be higher than generally appreciated because of inadequate examination of these two structures.

Involvement of the epicardium (visceral pericardium) and mural endocardium by granulomas usually represents an extension of the myocardial involvement into these layers of the heart. None of our patients or those previously described had epicardial or mural endocardial involvement without concomitant myocardial sarcoid granulomas. The occurrence of sarcoid granulomas in the adipose tissue adjacent to the coronary arteries, particularly the atrioventricular sulci, however, is unusual, whereas this portion of the heart is the area most frequently invaded by metastatic neoplasm [65–67]. Although their occurrence on the mediastinal aspect of the parietal pericardium is common, the occurrence of sarcoid granulomas on the cardiac (serous) aspect of the parietal pericardium is unusual. Such an occurrence, however, was observed in each of our two patients with recurring pericardial effusions. Rarely, valvular endocardium may contain sarcoid granulomas: in one of our 35 patients these granulomas were present on the pulmonic valve cusps, but they were not of sufficient size to cause valvular malfunction. Sarcoid involvement of the tricuspid valve has also been reported [39].

Whether or not cardiac dysfunction occurs as a consequence of cardiac sarcoidosis is dependent on at least three factors: (1) the number of sarcoid granulomas in the heart, i.e., the amount of ventricular myocardium replaced by granulomas versus the amount of uninvolved ventricular myocardium; (2) the amount of ventricular wall scarring, i.e., the amount of ventricular myocardium replaced by scar versus the amount of uninvolved ventricular myocardium, and (3) the location of the granulomas or scars within the heart. Of our 26 patients in whom cardiac dysfunction resulted from cardiac sarcoid (Table I), 23 had large, granulomas or scars on the left ventricular wall: two had recurring pericardial effusions and sarcoid granulomas in the pericardium, and one had a scar in the most cephalad portion of ventricular septum resulting in complete heart block. The amount of myocardium replaced by sarcoid granulomas was minute in each of our nine patients who had cardiac sarcoidosis and no cardiac dysfunction as a result of the cardiac granulomas (Table II). Indeed, in eight of these nine patients the cardiac granulomas were observed only by histologic examination. This also was the situation in the 15 patients described by others as having cardiac sarcoidosis but no cardiac dysfunction as a result of that infiltration (Table II).

The types of cardiac dysfunction produced by cardiac sarcoidosis include: (1) arrhythmias, primarily ventricular ones; (2) high degrees of atrioventricular block and complete bundle branch block; (3) sudden death; (4) congestive cardiac failure; (5) papillary muscle dysfunction; (6) "acute myocardial infarction"; (7) ventricular aneurysm and (8) recurring pericardial effusion.

Other than premature ventricular beats, ventricular tachycardia was the most frequent major arrhythmia, occurring in at least six (23 per cent) of our 26 patients (group IA) and in at least 12 (19 per cent) of 63 previously described patients with cardiac dysfunction resulting from cardiac sarcoidosis (group IIA). The occurrence of ventricular tachycardia in these patients usually indicates extensive sarcoid granulomatous involvement of the heart or extensive scarring as a result of healing of the granulomas. Atrial arrhythmias, present in four (15 per cent) patients in group IA and in 11 (17 per cent) of the 63 patients in group IIA did not appear to be direct consequences of cardiac sarcoidosis because only two of the 15 patients with atrial arrhythmias had sarcoid granulomas in the atrial walls at necropsy. The atrial arrhythmias more likely were consequences of atrial dilatation arising as a result of the ventricular malfunction.

Severe conduction disturbances also were common. Complete heart block was documented in six (23 per cent) patients in group IA and in 19 (30 per cent) of the 63 patients in group IIA. Of the 25 patients with complete heart block, 17 (68 per cent) also had episodes of syncope (Stokes-Adams attacks). In each of our five patients and in most if not all of the 19 previously described patients with complete heart block, the cephalad portion of the muscular ventricular septum, and especially that portion in the vicinity of the atrioventricular bundle, was extensively infiltrated by sarcoid granulomas or, in one patient, by scar tissue. In our one patient with complete heart block in whom serial histologic sections of the atrioventricular node and bundle were examined, partial destruction of the atrioventricular bundle and complete disruption of the bundle branches from their origin were observed. Similar observations have been made by Morales and associates [33]. Thus, complete heart block in these patients appears to result from interruption of the conduction pathways by either sarcoid granuloma or scar or both.

Complete bundle branch block also was common. It occurred in three (12 per cent) of our patients (group IA) and in 20 (32 per cent) of the patients in group IIA. The bundle branch block was right in 13, left in five and indeterminate in five. The patients with bundle branch block also had either granulomas or scars in the cephalad portion of the ventricular septum, but the amount of granulomatous or scar tissue appeared to be less extensive than that in patients with complete heart block.

Sudden death is the most common cardiac manifestation of clinically significant cardiac sarcoidosis. It occurred in 17 (65 per cent) of the patients in group IA and in 43 (68 per cent) of the patients in group IIA. That the sudden death in these 60 patients was of cardiac origin cannot be unequivocally proved, but many had had preceding arrhythmias or complete heart block, and ventricular fibrillation was confirmed terminally in several of them. Thus, sarcoidosis is an important but neglected cause of sudden cardiac death. Sudden death may be the initial manifestation of sarcoidosis. This was the case in six (35 per cent) of our 17 patients who died suddenly and in four (9 per cent) of the 43 previously described patients who died suddenly. Among these 10 patients (age range, 18 to 53 years [average 31]), death occurred during exertion in eight, and, although none had had symptoms, one had had ventricular premature beats documented by electrocardiogram. Of the remaining 50 patients who died suddenly, complete heart block had been present in 20 (40 per cent), ventricular tachycardia in 12 (24 per cent), ventricular premature beats in 11 (22 per cent) and atrial arrhythmias in seven (14 per cent). Of the 50 patients who died suddenly (excluding the 10 in whom sudden death was the initial manifestation of sarcoidosis), either complete heart block or a ventricular arrhythmia had been documented by electrocardiogram in 38 (76 per cent); of the remaining 12 patients, four had atrial arrhythmias, one had complete right bundle branch block, and seven never had an electrocardiogram recorded. Thus, ventricular arrhythmias and complete heart block are bad omens in patients with sarcoidosis.

Congestive cardiac failure is another common form of cardiac dysfunction in patients with extensive cardiac

TABLE VI Cardiac Sarcoidosis: Cardiac Aneurysm

Case No.	Reference	Age (yr)	Sex	Precordial Murmur	CHF	CHB	VT	SD	Length of Illness (mo)	CS Rx	Length of CS Rx (mo)	Site of Aneurysm RV	Site of Aneurysm LV	Myocardial Granuloma	Myocardial Transmural Scarring	Heart Weight (g)
1	Hines, Sancetta [19]	44	F	+	+	0	0	+	17	+	3	+	+	0	+	465
2	Duvernoy, Garcia [29]	30	F	+	+	0	+	+	30	+	—	0	+	+	—	—
3	Morales et al. [33]	41	M	—	—	0	0	+	—	—	—	0	+	+	—	—
4	Chun et al. [34]	49	F	+	—	0	+	+	38	+	30	0	+	0	+	470
5	Clark, Blount [44]	28	M	+	+	0	0	0	12	+	—	+	0	+	+	650
6	Freiman [46]	37	M	+	+	0	0	0	96	+	24	+	0	0	+	700
7	Present study	21	M	—	0	—	—	+	0	0	—	0	+	+	0	400
8	Present study	41	F	—	0	—	—	+	0	0	—	0	+	+	0	300

NOTE: 0 = absent; + = present; — = no information available; CHB = complete heart block; CHF = congestive heart failure; CS Rx = corticosteroid treatment; LV = left ventricle; RV = right ventricle; SD = sudden death; VT = ventricular tachycardia.

sarcoidosis. It occurred in eight (31 per cent) (fatal in six) of the patients in group IA and in 27 (43 per cent) (fatal in 14) of the patients in group IIA. With rare exception these 35 patients with congestive cardiac failure had extensive granulomas or scars in the left ventricular free wall, with or without similar involvement of the ventricular septum. The patients with congestive failure, however, had varying clinical features. In some, consequences of complete heart block or ventricular tachycardia dominated the clinical course and the failure was episodic. Most patients, however, had chronic failure.

Precordial systolic murmurs may be consequences of cardiac sarcoidosis. They were noted in four (15 per cent) of the patients in group IA and in 12 (19 per cent) [10,16,17,19,29,32,34,37,43,46,50] of the patients in group IIA. The murmurs usually were apical in location and varied from grade 1 to 5 (on a scale of 6) in intensity. Cardiac catheterization was performed in five patients [19,29,34,43,46] with precordial murmurs; in each of the four patients [19,29,43,46] in whom pulmonary arterial pressures were recorded, mild to moderate pulmonary hypertension was present and in one [43] the pulmonary arterial wedge pressure was greatly increased (v waves to 66 mm Hg). The cause of the murmurs in most of the 16 patients is unclear, but papillary muscle dysfunction is the most likely explanation. Although sarcoid granulomas in papillary muscle were described at necropsy in 29 (33 per cent) of the 89 patients in group IIA (no mention of papillary muscle in at least 27 patients) with cardiac dysfunction from cardiac sarcoidosis, precordial murmurs had been recorded in only six of them. Conversely, of the 16 patients with precordial murmurs, in only six (38 per cent) were sarcoid granulomas noted in their left ventricular papillary muscles at necropsy. Thus, although sarcoid infiltration into one or both left ventricular papillary muscles and into the free walls beneath them may produce papillary muscle dysfunction with mitral regurgitation, more often, the presence of a precordial murmur in these patients is not indicative of sarcoid in these structures. More often, the murmurs appear to result from altered papillary muscle dynamics due to dilatation of the left ventricle.

Ventricular aneurysm may be a consequence of cardiac sarcoidosis. A ventricular aneurysm occurred in two (8 per cent) of the patients in group IA and in six (10 per cent) of the patients in group IIA (Table VI). The aneurysm may involve either or both ventricular walls; it may be discrete and relatively small in the left ventricle, as illustrated by the patient described by Chun and associates [34] (Figure 10), or it may be diffuse and involve a large portion of the right ventricular wall, as occurred in the patient described by Freiman [46] (Figure 11) and in the patient described by Clark and

Blount [44]. Scarring or thinning of the ventricular septum may be associated with protrusion of the septum toward the right ventricle, producing, in effect, an internal cardiac aneurysm. Such was the probable case in the patient described by Hines and Sancetta [19]. The aneurysmal wall may or may not contain sarcoid granulomas: of the eight patients with ventricular aneurysms from cardiac sarcoidosis whose data are summarized in Table III, five had residual granulomas in the heart and three had none. In each of the latter three patients, the aneurysmal wall consisted entirely of fibrous tissue. The dominant component of the aneurysmal wall, however, in the other five patients also appears to have been fibrous tissue. The myocardial scarring and aneurysmal formation in these patients may have been related in part to the administration of corticosteroids. Of the 89 patients in groups IA and IIA, only nine (seven previously described [15,19,22,27,29,34,46]) had received corticosteroid therapy for longer than one month, and five of these nine patients were among the eight with ventricular aneurysms. The eight patients with ventricular aneurysms were young (range 21 to 49 years [average 36 years]). In only one [29] was the presence of a ventricular aneurysm recognized during life (by left ventricular angiography). Six of the eight patients died suddenly, and in two sudden death was the initial manifestation of sarcoidosis; the other two patients died of progressive congestive cardiac failure, and it is likely that their ventricular aneurysms contributed to, or were responsible for, the congestive failure. None of the eight patients had significant coronary arterial luminal narrowing. The occurrence of either right or left ventricular aneurysm in the absence of significant coronary arterial luminal narrowing is quite suggestive of cardiac sarcoidosis (which may or may not have "healed").

Excision of a left ventricular aneurysm of sarcoid origin at times may be beneficial. Lull and associates [68] described such an aneurysm, "the size of a tennis ball," which was resected in a 22 year old man with evidence of sarcoidosis for five months. Preoperatively, the patient had had episodes of ventricular tachycardia unresponsive to therapy with corticosteroids or antiarrhythmic agents. After aneurysmectomy, the ventricular arrhythmia, at the time of the report, was "no longer a problem." Although histologic examination of the wall of the resected aneurysm disclosed mainly fibrous tissue, a few sarcoid-type granulomas were present.

Although an effusion into a body cavity is an unusual feature of sarcoidosis, recurring pericardial effusion on occasion may be a prominent clinical manifestation of cardiac sarcoidosis. Such was the case in two (8 per cent) of the patients in group IA and in one (2 per cent) [47] patient in group IIA. A living patient with recurrent pericardial effusion secondary to pericardial sarcoidosis also was described by Shiff and associates [69]. This patient, a 31 year old woman, had a 1,000 ml serous effusion and multiple sarcoid granulomas on the epicardium. A possibly similar patient was described by Bailey [70]. The three necropsy patients were 27, 35 and 47 years of age, respectively, and two were women. Each had huge cardiac silhouettes typical of pericardial effusion. Two underwent thoracotomy shortly before death because of cardiac tamponade from large (800 ml each) pericardial effusions. At necropsy two of the three patients also had severe pulmonary sarcoidosis with considerable right ventricular hypertrophy, but the third had no sarcoid granulomas in the lung. Pericardial adhesions were present in one patient. All three had epicardial sarcoid granulomas; in addition, two had large and one had minute myocardial granulomas. Marked dilatation of both ventricles secondary to active or healed myocardial sarcoidosis may produce a "water-bottle" configuration of the cardiac silhouette on chest roentgenogram and mimic a large pericardial effusion. This situation occurred in the patient described by Clark and Blount [44]. Their patient proved to have only a small pericardial effusion but aneurysmal dilatation of both cardiac ventricles.

Because of its ability to cause arrhythmias, conduction disturbances, precordial murmurs, huge cardiac silhouettes, ventricular aneurysm and electrocardiographic evidence of "myocardial damage," cardiac sarcoidosis may mimic other cardiac conditions. In at least eight (31 per cent) of the patients in group IA and in five (8 per cent) [9,18,19,25,36] of the patients in group IIA, the initial clinical diagnosis was "acute myocardial infarction." The myocardial damage evident on the electrocardiogram may be the consequence of a sudden arrhythmia or complete heart block, or it may result entirely from the replacement of myocardium by sarcoid granulomas. Chest pain simulating acute myocardial infarction also was described in a patient described by Stephen [9] and in another described by Forbes and Usher [18]. Electrocardiograms were not diagnostic of, but compatible with, acute myocardial infarction in both patients; if necropsy had not been performed, coronary heart disease would have remained their diagnosis. Papillary muscle dysfunction in cardiac sarcoidosis may mimic valvular heart disease. The presentation of features of congestive cardiac failure associated with a large cardiac silhouette obviously may mimic idiopathic dilated cardiomyopathy [71] as well as pericardial effusion. The occurrence of very dilated ventricular cavities, particularly when associated with intracardiac thrombi, may even suggest this diagnosis at necropsy. Five of the 89 analyzed patients with cardiac dysfunction from cardiac sarcoidosis (groups IA and IIA) had intracardiac thrombi at

TABLE VII Cardiac Sarcoidosis: Effect of Corticosteroid Therapy on the Cardiac Granulomas

Case No.	Reference	Age (yr)	Sex	VT	CHB	CHF	Length of Illness (mo)	Length of CS Rx (mo)	SD	Cardiac Granulomas				Heart Weight (g)	No. of Cardiac Granulomas	Cardiac Aneurysm	
										LV	VS	RV	Atria			RV	LV
1	Porter [15]	19	M	0	+	0	24	7	+	+	+	+	—	—	—	0	0
2	Hines, Sancetta [19]	44	F	0	0	+	17	3	+	0	0	0	0	465	Few	0	+
3	Johansen [22]	43	M	0	+	0	108	108	+	0	+*	0	0	500	Few	0	0
4	Bashour et al. [27]	48	F	+	0	+	10	9	+	+	+	—	—	500	Few	0	0
5	Duvernoy, Garcia [29]	30	F	+	0	+	31	7	+	+	—	—	—	—	Few	0	+
6	Chun et al. [34]	49	F	+	0	—	38	30	+	0	0	0	0	470	0	0	+
7	Freiman [46]	37	M	0	0	+	96	24	0	0	0	0	0	700	0	+	0
8	Present study	30	M	+	0	0	53	7	+	+	+	+	0	450	Few	0	0
9	Present study	34	M	0	+	0	48	36	0	0	0	0	0	310	0	0	0

NOTE: 0 = absent; + = present; — = no information available; * = microscopic-sized; CHB = complete heart block; CHF = congestive heart failure; CS Rx = corticosteroid treatment; LV = left ventricle; RV = right ventricle; SD = sudden death; VS = ventricular septum; VT = ventricular tachycardia.

necropsy; four of the five had had severe congestive cardiac failure.

Another type of cardiac involvement in some patients with sarcoidosis is calcification of the mitral anulus. Although ectopic and metastatic calcification is a well recognized occurrence in patients with sarcoidosis [72,73,83], calcification of the mitral anulus has not been described previously in this condition. Nevertheless, one of the conditions which predisposes to mitral anular calcification is hypercalcemia, irrespective of its cause [74,75]. Because hypercalcemia is a recognized manifestation of sarcoidosis, it therefore is reasonable to believe that mitral anular calcification should occur with increased frequency in this condition. We found minimal deposits of calcium in the mitral anulus in one of our 35 patients with cardiac sarcoidosis (group I). This man was only 34 years of age, but he had severe hypercalcemia [76]. We found heavy mitral anular calcific deposits in another patient (not included in this study) who also had severe hypercalcemia from sarcoidosis but no cardiac sarcoid granulomas or myocardial scars (Figure 12). Both of these patients also received corticosteroid therapy for several years, and this medication possibly might also predispose to mitral anular calcification.

The effect of corticosteroid therapy on patients with cardiac sarcoid granulomas has received little attention. Analysis of the data on our and previously described necropsy patients with cardiac sarcoidosis strongly suggests that this medication promotes healing of the cardiac granulomas. Only three of the patients in group IA and only 12 of the patients in group IIA received corticosteroid therapy at some time; only nine of these 15 patients received this medication for longer than one month. Certain clinical and morphologic observations in them are summarized in Table VII. Of these nine patients, four had no sarcoid granulomas in the heart—only myocardial scars at sites preferentially involved by sarcoid—and each of the remaining five patients had mainly myocardial scars with relatively few residual granulomas. The four patients without any cardiac granulomas were the only ones among the entire group of 113 patients (Tables II through IV) who had no cardiac granulomas, and three of the four also had one or more cardiac aneurysms at sites of myocardial scarring. Only one of the eight patients with a cardiac aneurysm had not received corticosteroid therapy. Thus, the evidence is substantial that corticosteroid therapy can cause healing of cardiac granulomas but that a possible consequence of this healing is the development of a cardiac aneurysm (Figure 13). The administration of corticosteroids over a period of several weeks during acute myocardial infarction resulting from severe coronary atherosclerosis also can lead rapidly to the development of a cardiac aneurysm [77].

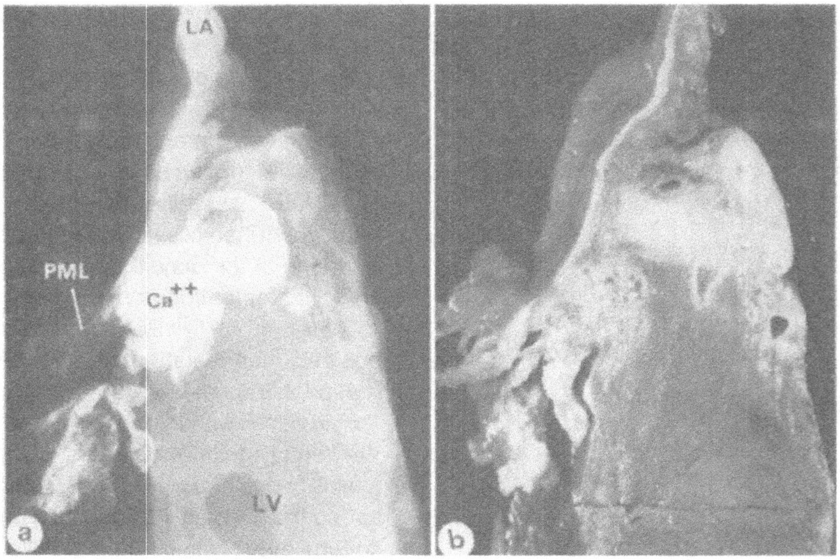

*Figure 12. Longitudinal cut of left atrium (LA), posterior mitral leaflet (PML) and left ventricle (LV) in a 44 year old black woman (A75-12) who had had evidence of noncardiac sarcoidosis for 18 years. Hypercalcemia developed and she died from rupture of a peptic ulcer, apparently a consequence of corticosteroid therapy. A surprise finding at necropsy was the presence of large calcific deposits (Ca++) in the mitral anular region as shown here. A tongue of calcium also protruded from the anular area into the space just behind the posterior mitral leaflet. Hypercalcemia, and possibly also prolonged corticosteroid therapy, are precursors to mitral anular calcification. **a**, roentgenogram. **b**, specimen itself.*

Indirect evidence that corticosteroid therapy causes "shrinkage" of the cardiac sarcoid granulomas is demonstrated by the reported diminution in the frequency of arrhythmias, conduction disturbances and electrocardiographic evidence of myocardial damage after initiation of this medication [78–81].

Sarcoid granulomas in the heart may be more responsive to corticosteroid therapy than are sarcoid granulomas located in other body organs. Of the four patients with no residual cardiac sarcoid granulomas, only one [46] had no residual granulomas in other body organs at necropsy. (Lymph node biopsy in the patient before he was given corticosteroid therapy had disclosed many sarcoid granulomas.) Of the other five patients with few cardiac sarcoid granulomas, all appeared to have relatively larger numbers of granulomas in other body organs. Obviously, a possible explanation for this observation is that the area for sarcoid granulomatous infiltration is larger in the liver or lung than in the heart; in other words, the area for granulomatous

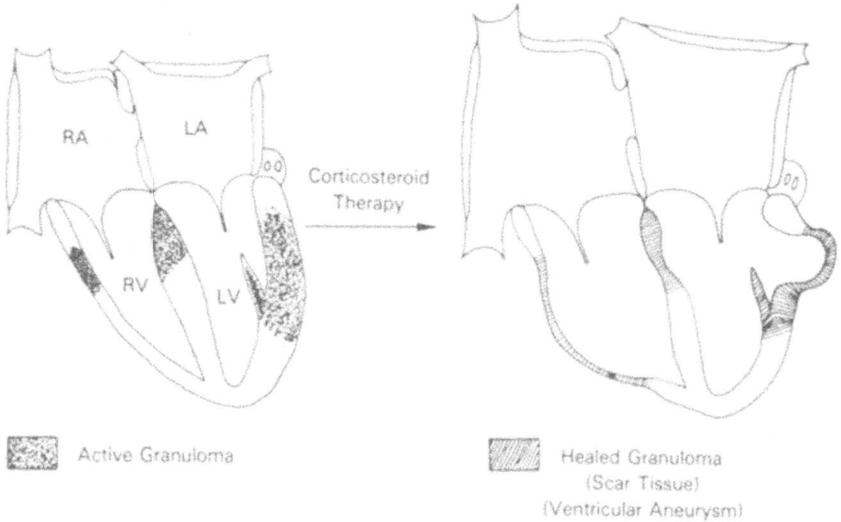

Figure 13. Diagram showing the good and bad effects of corticosteroid therapy in patients with cardiac sarcoidosis.

infiltration in the heart is smaller than that of some other body organs.

The majority of patients, in whom cardiac sarcoidosis causes cardiac dysfunction, present initially with manifestations related to the heart rather than to involvement of other body organs or systems. The initial manifestation of sarcoidosis in 23 (88 per cent) of the patients in group IA was related to the heart. Among the previously described 63 patients (group IIA), information regarding the initial manifestation was available in 38: in 28 (74 per cent) of them the initial manifestation was related to signs or symptoms of cardiac dysfunction. Furthermore, in the majority of these 89 patients (26 plus 63) there was never any clinical evidence of dysfunction of an organ system other than the heart. Indeed, the occurrence of symptomatic involvement of another body system by sarcoid generally indicates that symptom-producing cardiac involvement by sarcoid is unlikely to occur. Fleming [80], in search of patients with cardiac sarcoid, surveyed the chest, eye and skin clinics in his hospital in which patients with other forms of sarcoidosis were being followed and found this search unprofitable in revealing patients with cardiac sarcoid. Thus, cardiac sarcoidosis severe enough to cause cardiac dysfunction tends to be an all or none process: if it causes cardiac dysfunction, it tends not to cause dysfunction of another organ system; conversely, if it causes dysfunction of a noncardiac organ system, it infrequently causes cardiac dysfunction.

Although signs or symptoms of cardiac dysfunction from cardiac sarcoidosis may be present for many years, more often the course is not prolonged. The duration of symptoms of cardiac dysfunction from cardiac sarcoidosis was 12 months or less in 19 (73 per cent) of the patients in group IA and in 26 (58 per cent) of the 45 previously described patients (information not available in 18) in group IIA.

Although it appears to be the major cause of giant cell myocarditis, sarcoidosis is not the only condition in which giant cells unassociated with stainable organisms occur in the heart. Giant cells also have been observed in the hearts of patients with infective endocarditis [82], rheumatoid arthritis [83], Takayasu's arteritis [84], Wegener's granulomatosis [85] and, rarely, in patients with coronary heart disease with or without systemic hypertension [71]. "Idiopathic" granulomatous (giant cell) myocarditis has been reported by a number of investigators [86–94], but in many such reports the condition described may not have been "isolated" and, therefore, almost surely [86–90] or probably [91–94] was **cardiac sarcoidosis.** If the latter condition is defined as the presence of "hard" granulomas in at least one other body organ (always lymph node) in addition to the heart, then many patients described as having "isolated" giant cell or granulomatous myocarditis in actuality had cardiac sarcoidosis. It is probable that many patients reported to have isolated granulomatous (giant cell) myocarditis also had giant cells in lymph nodes but that these structures were not examined histologically. In several described patients and in a few of our patients with cardiac sarcoidosis, the lymph nodes were not enlarged grossly; if the nodes had not been studied histologically, sarcoidosis would not have been diagnosed. Thus, a diagnosis of "isolated granulomatous (giant cell) myocarditis" is justified only after thorough exclusion of extracardiac sarcoidosis. In contrast to Davies et al. [90], we believe that "idiopathic giant cell myocarditis" and "cardiac sarcoidosis" cannot be distinguished by histologic examination of the heart alone.

REFERENCES

1. Brosig W: Zur tuberkulösen Erkrankung des Herzmuskels. Zentralbl Allg Pathol 72: 161, 1939.
2. Longcope WT, Fisher AM: The effect of Schaumann's disease upon the heart and its mechanism. Acta Med Scand 108: 529, 1941.
3. Bates GS, Walsh JM: Boeck's sarcoid: observations on seven patients, one autopsy. Ann Intern Med 29: 306, 1948.
4. Scotti TM, McKeown CE: Sarcoidosis involving the heart. Report of case with sudden death. Arch Pathol 46: 289, 1948.
5. Vogt H: Morbus Besnier-Boeck-Schaumann. Klinische und pathologische-anatomie Studie. Helv Med Acta 16 (suppl 25): 1, 1949.
6. Kulka WE: Sarcoidosis of the heart. A cause of sudden and unexpected death. Circulation 1: 772, 1950.
7. Simkins S: Boeck's sarcoid with complete heart block mimicking carotid sinus syncope. Report of a case. JAMA 146: 794, 1951.
8. Oille WA, Ritchie RC, Barrie HJ: The age of lesions in a case of myocardial sarcoidosis. Can Med Assoc J 68: 277, 1953.
9. Stephen JD: Fatal myocardial sarcoidosis. A case of sudden death. Circulation 9: 886, 1954.
10. Powell LW Jr: Sarcoidosis of the myocardium. NC Med J 15: 28, 1954.
11. Gottfarb AG, Wahlgren F: Adams-Stokes syndrom framkallat av morbus Besnier-Boeck-Schaumann (sarcoidosis). Nord Med 52: 985, 1954.
12. Clinicopathologic conference. Cardiac arrhythmia. US Armed Forces Med J 8: 855, 1957.
13. Peacock RA, Lippschutz EJ, Lukas A: Myocardial sarcoidosis. Circulation 16: 67, 1957.
14. Poon TP, Forbus WD: Sudden death due to myocardial sarcoidosis, with a comment on the etiology of sarcoid. Arch Intern Med 104: 771, 1959.
15. Porter GH: Sarcoid heart disease. N Engl J Med 263: 1350, 1960.
16. Phinney AO Jr: Sarcoid of the myocardial septum with complete heart block. Report of two cases. Am Heart J 62: 270, 1961.
17. Chamovitz DL, Culley AW, Carlson KE: Cardiac sarcoidosis. Report of a case with paroxysmal ventricular tachycardia.

JAMA 182: 574, 1962.
18. Forbes G, Usher A: Fatal myocardial sarcoidosis. Br Med J 2: 771, 1962.
19. Hines JD, Sancetta SM: Myocardial sarcoidosis simulating healed myocardial infarction. Ohio State Med J 59: 689, 1963.
20. Smith WP: Primary sarcoid heart disease. Report of a case. J Fla Med Assoc 51: 652, 1964.
21. Chomette G, Auriol M, Daddi G, et al.: Localisations cardiaques massives d'une sarcoïdose de Besnier-Boeck-Schaumann. Ann Anat Pathol (Paris) 10: 177, 1965.
22. Johansen A: Isolated myocarditis versus myocardial sarcoidosis. A contribution to the discussion regarding points of resemblance between these and a report of three illustrative cases. Acta Pathol Microbiol Scand 67: 15, 1966.
23. Shimada N, Ishihara Y, Kojima A, et al.: Three cases of granulomatous myocarditis with giant cells. Acta Pathol Jap 17: 503, 1967.
24. Miyaji T, Ohara M, Funaki M, et al.: [A case of myocardial sarcoidosis with Adams-Stokes syndrome]. J Jap Soc Intern Med 56: 260, 1967.
25. Contreras R, Sánchez Torres G, Durán Rodríquez P: Sarcoidosis cardiaca. Arch Inst Cardiol Mex 37: 20, 1967.
26. Hishimoto Y, Takano Y, Tagaki M: Case of fatal myocardial sarcoidosis preceded by cardiac symptoms. Jap J Clin Med 26: 1244, 1968.
27. Bashour FA, McConnell T, Skinner W, et al.: Myocardial sarcoidosis. Dis Chest 53: 413, 1968.
28. Rajasenan V, Cooper ES: Myocardial sarcoidosis, bouts of ventricular tachycardia, psychiatric manifestations and sudden death. A case report. J Natl Med Assoc 61: 306, 1969.
29. Duvernoy WFC, Garcia R: Sarcoidosis of the heart presenting with ventricular tachycardia and atrioventricular block. Am J Cardiol 28: 348, 1971.
30. Rossi L: Sarcoid heart disease. Br Med J 1: 546, 1973.
31. Ghosh P, Fleming HA, Gresham GA, et al.: Myocardial sarcoidosis. Br Heart J 34: 769, 1972.
32. Zoneraich S, Gupta MP, Mehta J, et al.: Myocardial sarcoidosis presenting as acute mitral insufficiency. Chest 66: 452, 1974.
33. Morales AR, Levy S, Davis J, et al.: Sarcoidosis and the heart. Pathology Annual 1974 (Sommers SC, ed), New York, Appleton-Century-Crofts, 1974, p 139.
34. Chun SK, Andy JJ, Jilly P, et al.: Ventricular aneurysm in sarcoidosis. Chest 68: 392, 1975.
35. Johnson JB, Jason RS: Sarcoidosis of the heart. Report of a case and review of the literature. Am Heart J 27: 246, 1944.
36. Yesner R, Silver M: Fatal myocardial sarcoidosis. Am Heart J 41: 777, 1951.
37. Adickes GC, Zimmerman SL, Cardwell ES: Sarcoidosis with fatal cardiac involvement. Ann Intern Med 35: 898, 1951.
38. Arkless HA, Gokcebay TM, Mendell TH: Sarcoidosis of the heart. Am J Cardiol 1: 648, 1958.
39. Stein MH, Gross JM, Shulman H: A case of cardiac sarcoidosis manifested by uncontrollable ventricular tachycardia. Review of cardiac manifestations in sixteen cases of sarcoidosis. Am J Cardiol 10: 864, 1962.
40. Ferrans VJ, Hibbs RG, Black WC, et al.: Myocardial degeneration in cardiac sarcoidosis. Histochemical and electron microscopic studies. Am Heart J 68: 159, 1965.
41. Carvalhal S dos S, Rocha JC: Un caso de sarcoidose com comprometimento de coraçao. Rev Assoc Med Brasil 11: 89, 1965.
42. Deneberg M: Sarcoidosis of the myocardium and aorta. A case report. Am J Clin Pathol 43: 445, 1965.
43. Raftery EB, Oakley CM, Goodwin JF: Acute subvalvular mitral incompetence. Lancet 2: 360, 1966.
44. Clark EJ, Blount AW: A fatal case of myocardial sarcoidosis. Lancet 86: 568, 1966.
45. Bruno MS, Ober WB: Clinico-pathologic conference. Intractable heart failure with long-standing granulomatous disease. NY State J Med 68: 2790, 1968.
46. Case Records of the Massachusetts General Hospital. Case 46–1975. Harthorne JW, Freiman DG. N Engl J Med 293: 1138, 1975.
47. Gozo EG Jr, Cosnow I, Cohen HC, et al.: The heart in sarcoidosis. Chest 60: 379, 1971.
48. Cotter EF: Boeck's sarcoid. Autopsy in a case with visceral lesions. Arch Intern Med 64: 286, 1939.
49. Hirayama J: Ein Fall von diffuser spezifischer Myocarditis mit zahlreichen Riesenzellen. Trans Soc Pathol Jap 29: 261, 1939.
50. Botti RE, Young FE: Myocardial sarcoid, complete heart block and aortic stenosis. Ann Intern Med 51: 811, 1959.
51. Nissen AW, Berte JB: Cardiac arrhythmias in sarcoidosis. Arch Intern Med 113: 275, 1964.
52. Bernstein M, Konzlemann FW, Sidlick DM: Boeck's sarcoid. Report of a case with visceral involvement. Arch Intern Med 44: 721, 1929.
53. Nickerson DA: Boeck's sarcoid. Report of six cases in which autopsies were made. Arch Pathol 24: 19, 1937.
54. Spencer J, Warren S: Boeck's sarcoid. Report of a case, with clinical diagnosis confirmed at autopsy. Arch Intern Med 62: 285, 1938.
55. Granström KO, Gripwall E, Kristofferson CE, et al.: A case of uveoparotid fever (Heerfordt) with autopsy findings. Acta Med Scand 126: 307, 1946.
56. Skavlem JH, Ritterhoff RJ: Coexistent pulmonary asbestosis and sarcoidosis. Am J Pathol 22: 493, 1946.
57. Gendel BR, Young JM, Greiner DJ: Sarcoidosis. A review with twenty-four additional cases. Am J Med 12: 205, 1952.
58. Gilg I: Sarcoidosis involving the heart. Acta Derm Venereol 33: 318, 1953.
59. Brun J, Turiaf J, Perrin LF, et al.: Coeur et sarcoidose de Besnier-Boeck-Schaumann. Presse Med 63: 284, 1955.
60. Pascoe HR: Myocardial sarcoidosis. Report of a case with unexpected death. Arch Pathol 77: 299, 1964.
61. Peison B: Sarcoidosis of the heart associated with myocarditis: report of case. Ill Med J 130: 317, 1966.
62. Smith LH Jr: Case Records of the Massachusetts General Hospital. Weekly Clinicopathological Exercises. Case 8–1974. N Engl J Med 290: 504, 1974.
63. Laroche C, de Gennes J-L, Hazard J, et al.: Maladie de Besnier-Boeck-Schaumann avec manifestations polyarticulaires et localisations endo-myo-péricardiques mortelles. Bull Mém Soc Med Hôp Paris 71: 908, 1955.
64. Thorbjarnarson B, Glenn F: Sarcoidosis associated with sudden death during mitral valvulotomy. Arch Surg 73: 862, 1956.
65. Roberts WC, Bodey GP, Wertlake PT: The heart in acute leukemia. A study of 420 autopsy cases. Am J Cardiol 21: 388, 1968.
66. Glancy DL, Roberts WC: The heart in malignant melanoma. A study of 70 autopsy cases. Am J Cardiol 21: 555, 1968.
67. Roberts WC, Glancy DL, DeVita VT Jr: Heart in malignant lymphoma (Hodgkin's disease, lymphosarcoma, reticulum cell sarcoma and mycosis fungoides). A study of 196 autopsy cases. Am J Cardiol 22: 85, 1968.
68. Lull RJ, Dunn BE, Gregoratos G, et al.: Ventricular aneurysm due to cardiac sarcoidosis with surgical cure of refractory ventricular tachycardia. Am J Cardiol 30: 282, 1972.
69. Shiff AD, Blatt CJ, Colp C: Recurrent pericardial effusion secondary to sarcoidosis of the pericardium. A biopsy-proven case. N Engl J Med 281: 141, 1969.
70. Bailey RR: Systemic sarcoidosis with pericarditis and pericardial effusion. N Z Med J 65: 704, 1966.
71. Roberts WC, Ferrans VJ: Pathologic anatomy of the cardiomyopathies. Idiopathic dilated and hypertrophic types,

infiltrative types, and endomyocardial disease with and without eosinophilia. Hum Pathol 6: 287, 1975.
72. Lathan SR, Block RA, McLean RL: Sarcoidosis with metastatic calcification. Am J Med 44: 1000, 1968.
73. Fujita N, Torres A, Sharma OP: Ectopic calcification in sarcoidosis. JAMA 227: 556, 1974.
74. Roberts WC: Calcification of the mitral anulus: a study of 87 necropsy patients (abstract). Circulation 45 & 46 (Suppl II): 107, 1972.
75. Roberts WC, Perloff JK: Mitral valvular disease. A clinicopathologic survey of the conditions causing the mitral valve to function abnormally. Ann Intern Med 77: 939, 1972.
76. Bell NH, Bartter FC: Studies of ^{47}Ca metabolism in sarcoidosis: evidence for increased sensitivity of bone to vitamin D. Acta Endocrinol (Kbh) 54: 173, 1967.
77. Bulkley BH, Roberts WC: Steroid therapy during acute myocardial infarction. A cause of delayed healing and of ventricular aneurysm. Am J Med 56: 244, 1974.
78. Gold J, Cantor P: Sarcoid heart disease. A case with unusual electrocardiogram. Arch Intern Med 104: 101, 1959.
79. Unsigned Editorial. Myocardial sarcoidosis. Lancet 2: 1351, 1972.
80. Fleming HA: Sarcoid heart disease. Br Med J 1: 174, 1973.
81. Strauss GS, Lawton BR, Wenzel FJ, et al.: Detection of covert myocardial sarcoidosis by scalene node biopsy. Chest 69: 790, 1976.
82. Buchbinder NA, Roberts WC: Left-sided valvular active infective endocarditis. A study of forty-five necropsy patients. Am J Med 53: 20, 1972.
83. Roberts WC, Kehoe JA, Carpenter DF, et al.: Cardiac valvular lesions in rheumatoid arthritis. Arch Intern Med 122: 141, 1968.
84. Roberts WC, Wibin EA: Idiopathic panaortitis, supra-aortic arteritis, granulomatous myocarditis and pericarditis. A cause of pulseless disease and possibly left ventricular aneurysm in the African. Am J Med 41: 453, 1966.
85. Walton EW: Giant-cell granuloma of the respiratory tract (Wegener's granulomatosis). Br Med J 2: 265, 1958.
86. Jonas AF Jr: Granulomatous myocarditis. Bull Johns Hopkins Hosp 64: 45, 1939.
87. Kean BH, Koekenga MT: Giant cell myocarditis. Am J Pathol 28: 1095, 1952.
88. Tesluk H: Giant cell versus granulomatous myocarditis. Am J Clin Pathol 26: 1326, 1956.
89. Long WH: Granulomatous (Fiedler's) myocarditis with extracardiac involvement. A case report with sudden death. JAMA 177: 184, 1961.
90. Davies MJ, Pomerance A, Teare RD: Idiopathic giant cell myocarditis—a distinctive clinico-pathological entity. Br Heart J 37: 192, 1975.
91. Manger D: A case of fatal subacute myocarditis of unknown etiology. Am J Med Sci 198: 246, 1939.
92. Saphir O: Isolated myocarditis. Am Heart J 24: 167, 1942.
93. Dilling NV: Giant-cell myocarditis. J Pathol Bacteriol 71: 295, 1956.
94. Rab SM, Choudhury GM, Choudhury AR: Giant-cell myocarditis. Lancet 2: 172, 1963.

STRUCTURE — FUNCTION CORRELATIONS IN CARDIOVASCULAR AND PULMONARY DISEASES (CPC)

Cardiac Sarcoidosis*

A Major Cause of Sudden Death in Young Individuals

Renu Virmani, M.D.; J. Conrad Bures, M.D.; and William C. Roberts, M.D., F.C.C.P.

Dr. William C. Roberts: Herein we will discuss certain findings in a patient with cardiac sarcoidosis. Dr. Virmani will describe the patient.

Dr. Renu Virmani: A 35-year-old white man, a college philosophy professor who died Jan 9, 1979, was observed to have occasional ventricular premature beats during a medical check-up in March 1978 (ten months before death). No other abnormalities were found on examination. Specifically, he had no precordial murmur. He weighed 73.6 kg and was 175 cm tall. The ECG (Fig 1) showed low voltage, and chest roentgenogram (Fig 2) showed a normal sized heart and normal hilar and pulmonary shadows. In May 1978, he had an "upper respiratory infection," and in June 1978, he noted exertional dyspnea, two-pillow orthopnea, pedal edema, and severe fatigue.

*From the Pathology Branch, National Heart, Lung, and Blood Institute, National Institutes of Health, Bethesda, and the Department of Pathology, Montefiore Hospital, University of Pittsburgh Health Center, Pittsburgh.
Reprint requests: Dr. Roberts, NIH, Bldg 10A, Room 3E30, Bethesda 20205

He was hospitalized in July 1978, his first and only hospitalization. The blood pressure was 110/70 mm Hg. The jugular veins were distended; rales were heard over both lungs; the heart was enlarged; a grade 2/6 holosystolic murmur now was heard at the lower left sternal border and it increased with inspiration; a third heart sound was present; and the feet were edematous. The blood hematocrit value was 45 percent; white blood cell count, 10,200/cu mm; blood urea nitrogen value, 38 mg/100 ml; serum creatinine level, 1.4 mg/100 ml; and serum total cholesterol value, 126 mg/100 ml. The IgG immunoglobulins were "low." The ECG was similar to the preceding one. The echocardiogram disclosed the maximal dimensions of the left ventricle to be 70 mm (normal, 40 to 52; left atrium, 45 mm (normal, 15 to 35); and the aorta, 30 mm (normal, 20 to 35). The walls of both the left ventricle and ventricular septum were 10 mm thick. Catheterization on July 25, 1979, disclosed the following pressures (mm Hg): pulmonary arterial wedge mean, 28; a-wave, 30, v-wave, 44; pulmonary trunk, 55/30 (mean 40);

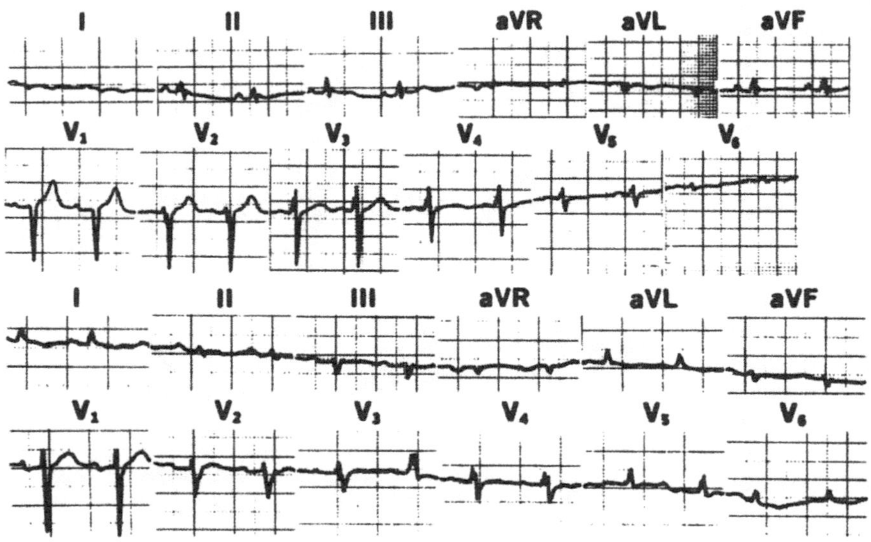

FIGURE 1. Electrocardiograms taken 3/6/78 (*upper*) and 9/6/78 (*lower*). Both show low voltage and nonspecific T-wave changes. One extrasystole is present in the lower electrocardiogram.

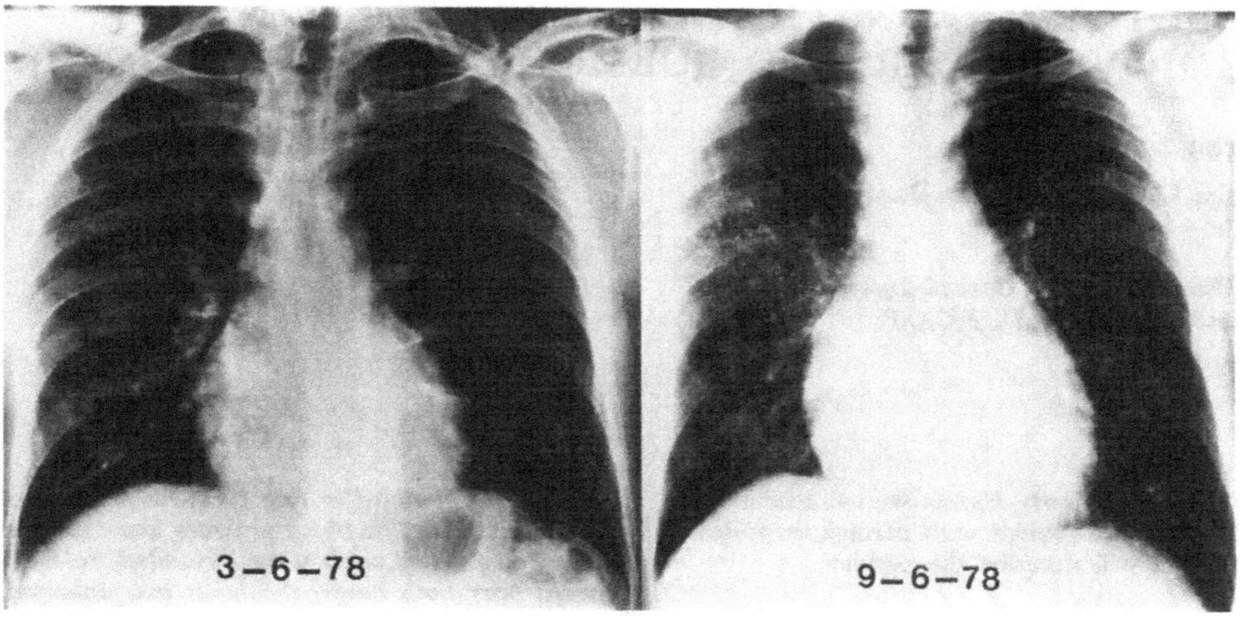

FIGURE 2. Chest roentgenograms taken 3/6/78 and 9/6/78. Cardiac silhouette has increased in size. Lung and hilar areas are normal.

right ventricle, 55/12; and right atrial mean, 10, a-wave 16. A diagnosis of idiopathic dilated cardiomyopathy was made and he was treated with digitalis, quinidine, chlorothiazide, and warfarin sodium. The dyspnea lessened considerably, the edema vanished, and he returned to his teaching duties. In September 1978, his weight was down to 146 pounds, his neck veins were flat, there was no edema, but a grade 3/6 murmur of tricuspid regurgitation persisted and a right ventricular lift was present. On Oct 13, 1978, he was started on a regimen of prednisone (10 mg daily), but during the next ten days, no subjective improvement was noted, and therefore, this medication was gradually discontinued over several more days. He remained asymptomatic until about Dec 20, 1978, when mild exertional dyspnea and orthopnea returned. His neck veins were distended, and the liver was both palpable and pulsatile. The weight had increased to 156 pounds, but he was not overtly edematous. He collapsed suddenly 19 days later while teaching and died.

Dr. Roberts: Dr. Bures, would you describe the findings at autopsy.

Dr. J. Conrad Bures: At necropsy (Montefiore Hospital, Pittsburgh), the heart weighed 460 g. All four cavities were dilated. The walls of both ventricles and both atria contained firm white deposits which histologically were typical sarcoid granulomas (Fig 3 to 6). The four cardiac valves and the coronary arteries were normal. Calcific deposits were present in a few myocardial fibers in the walls of all four cardiac chambers. The lungs together weighed 1,040 g; A 0.4-cm sized subpleural sarcoid granuloma was present in the right upper lobe. The tracheobronchial nodes measured up to 2 cm in diameter and they were nearly totally replaced by sarcoid granulomas (Fig 7). The liver (weight, 1,800 g) and spleen (weight, 300 g) were congested but free of granulomas. The rest of the organs were normal.

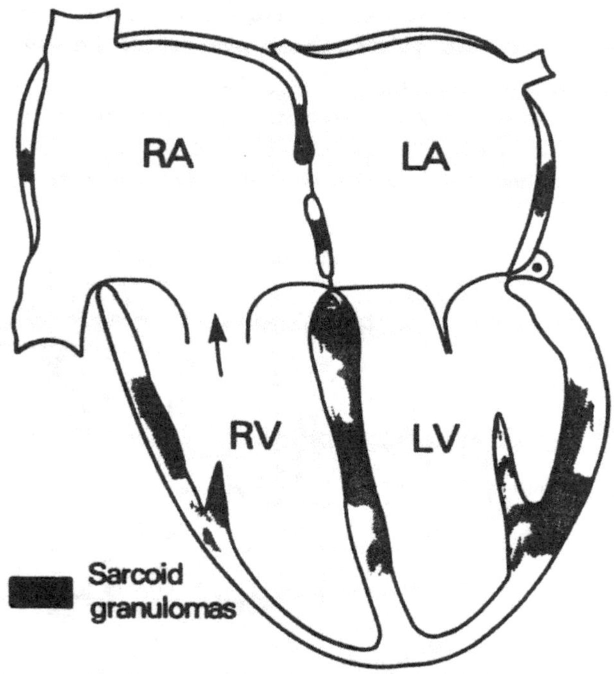

FIGURE 3. Diagram of heart at necropsy showing approximate location of sarcoid granulomas. RA indicates right atrium; RV, right ventricle; LA, left atrium; and LV, left ventricle.

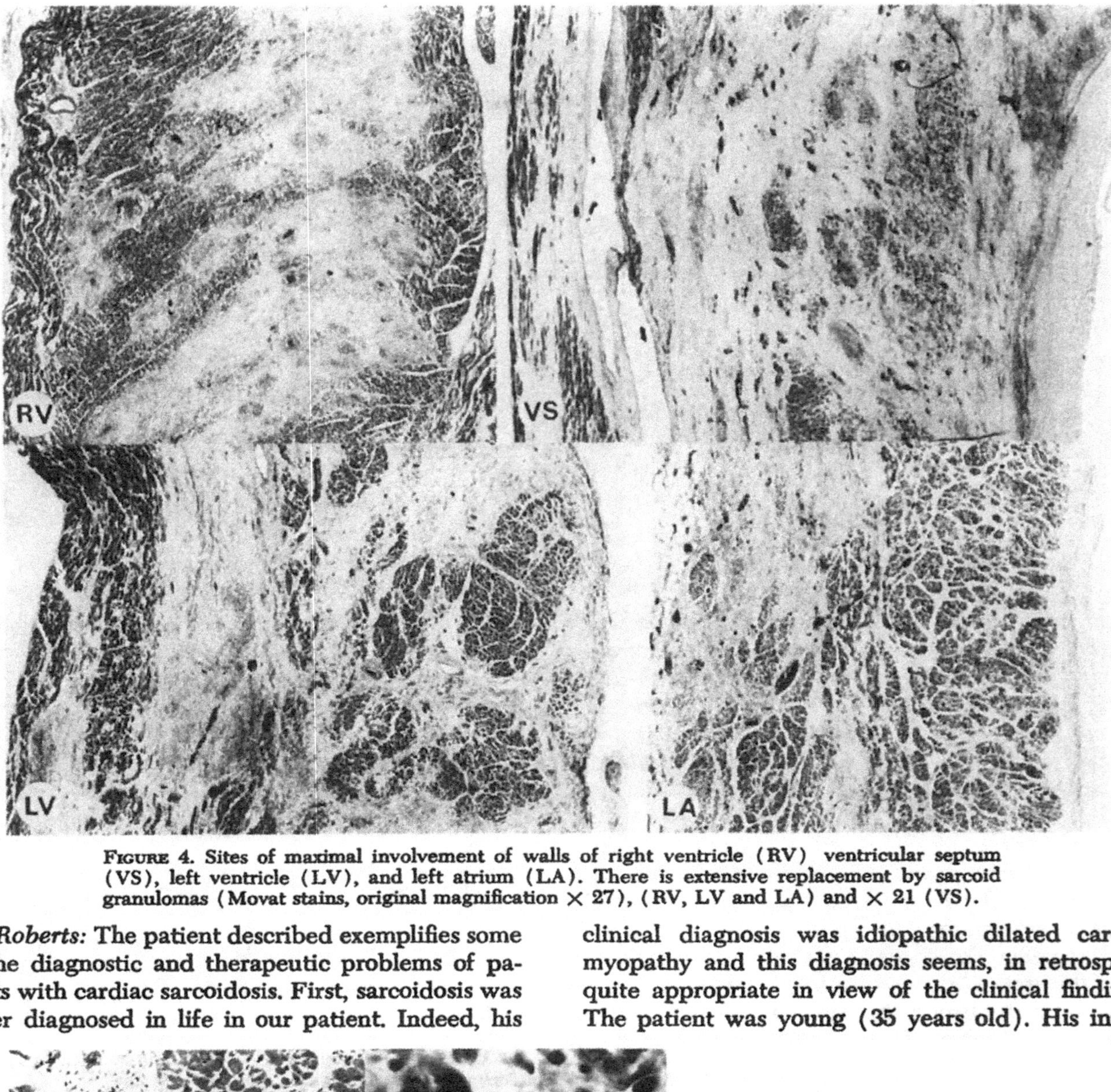

FIGURE 4. Sites of maximal involvement of walls of right ventricle (RV) ventricular septum (VS), left ventricle (LV), and left atrium (LA). There is extensive replacement by sarcoid granulomas (Movat stains, original magnification × 27), (RV, LV and LA) and × 21 (VS).

Dr. Roberts: The patient described exemplifies some of the diagnostic and therapeutic problems of patients with cardiac sarcoidosis. First, sarcoidosis was never diagnosed in life in our patient. Indeed, his clinical diagnosis was idiopathic dilated cardiomyopathy and this diagnosis seems, in retrospect, quite appropriate in view of the clinical findings. The patient was young (35 years old). His initial

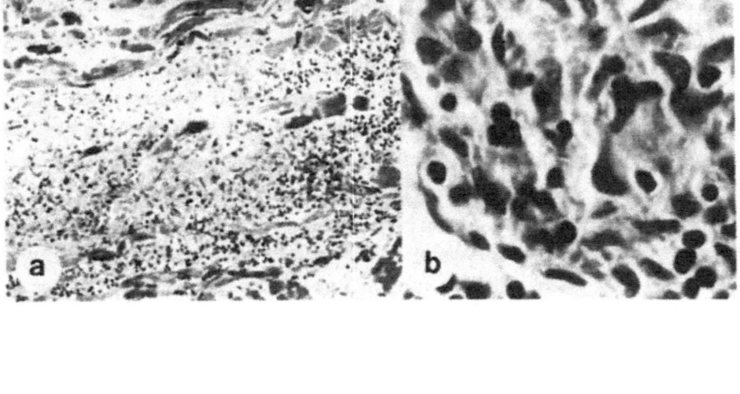

FIGURE 5. Extensive, sarcoid granulomatous involvement of left atrium. b (*right*), Close-up of giant cell, epitheloid cells and lymphocytes, a (*left*), Movat stain, original magnification × 130, and b (*right*), hematoxylin-eosin, original magnification × 880).

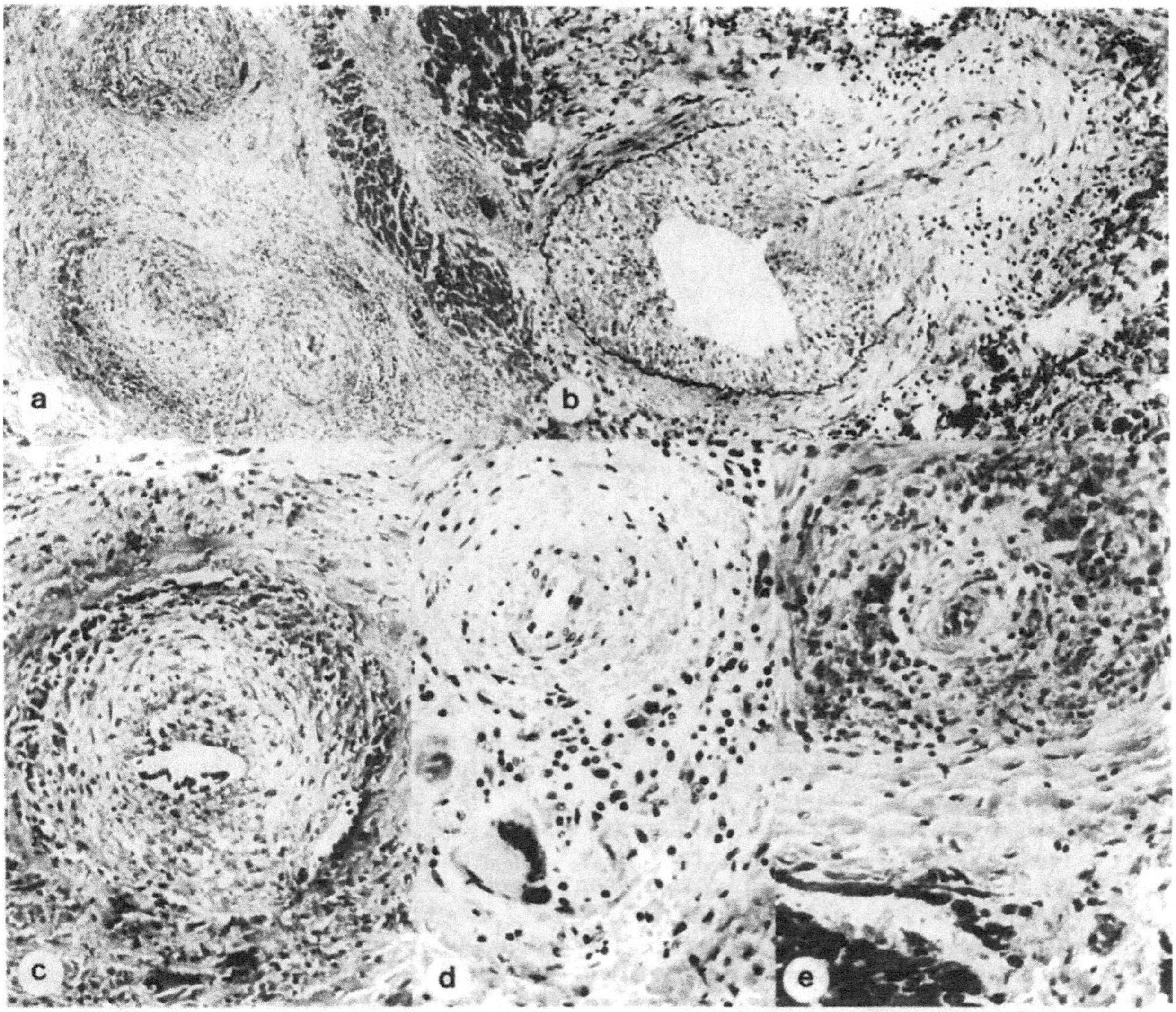

FIGURE 6. Intramural coronary arteries of ventricular septum, a, b, c, and d (*top figures* and *bottom, left* and *center*), and left ventricular free wall, e (*bottom right*) with surrounding sarcoid granulomas (sarcoid arteritis). Arteries or arterioles are surrounded by sarcoid granulomas and intima is thickened (Movat stains, original magnifications a [*top left*], × 80; b [*top right*], × 180; c [*bottom left*], × 220; d [*bottom center*], × 330; and e [*bottom right*, × 290]).

manifestation was ventricular premature beats which were noted on routine physical examination ten months before death, and he remained asymptomatic until six months before death when evidence of congestive heart failure appeared. He had cardiomegaly, a murmur of tricuspid regurgitation, and overt congestive heart failure which initially was quite responsive to medical therapy, but in his last month, reappeared. Because he was young and never had chest pain, coronary heart disease as a possibility never arose. The absence of a precordial murmur at the onset of his illness ruled out organic valvular heart disease as a reasonable diagnosis. During life, there were no signs suggesting the possibility of sarcoidosis. Chest roentgenogram showed normal lungs and no hilar adenopathy. Furthermore, lymph nodes were never palpated on physical examination. Moreover, there were no signs or symptoms of pulmonary disease. The mild hepatomegaly and splenomegaly were consistent with congestive heart failure and certainly did not suggest an infiltrative process, and at necropsy, no granulomas were present in either the liver or the spleen, and indeed, only one granuloma was observed in the lungs. There were no demonstrated ventricular arrhythmias other than an occasional ventricular premature beat during his illness. There were no cardiac conduction disturbances, heart block, syncope, or dizzy spells. Thus, clinically either retrospectively or prospectively, a diagnosis of sarcoidosis in the present patient would have been extremely difficult.

Approximately three months before death, the pa-

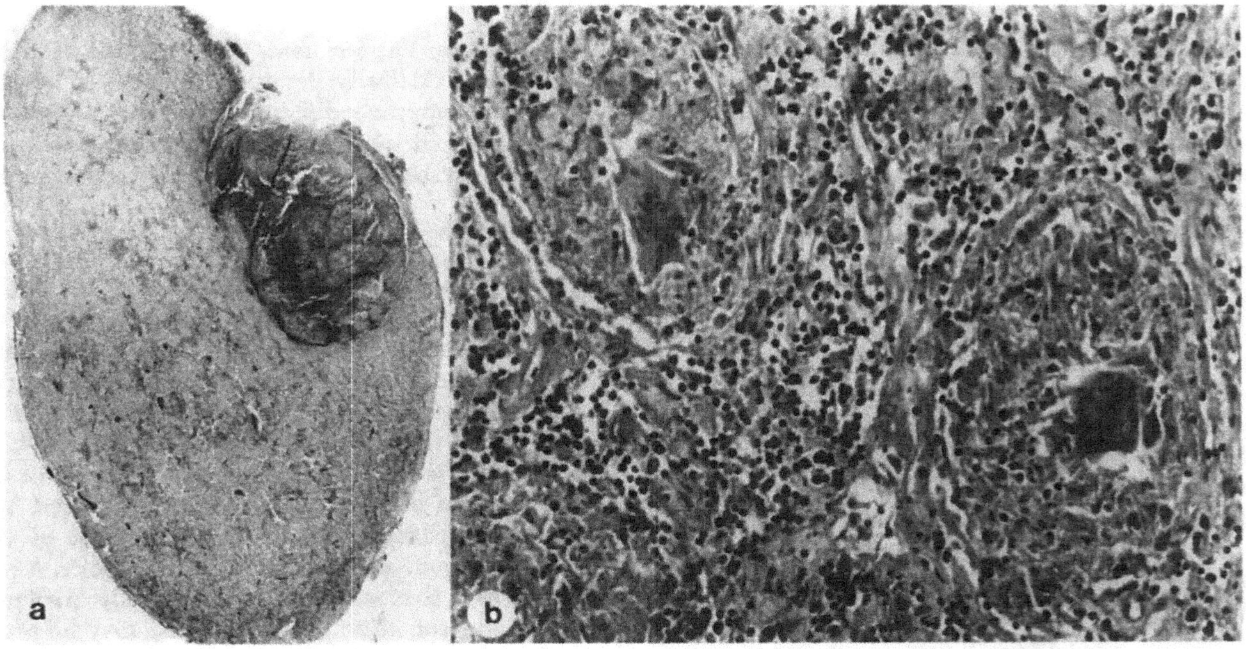

FIGURE 7. Tracheobronchial lymph node showing extensive replacement by sarcoid granulomas (hematoxylin-eosin, original magnificatoins a [*left*], × 8 and b [*right*], × 196]).

tient was given prednisone for about 15 days. Because no subjective improvement was noted, this medication was stopped. This patient brings up the possibility of a trial period of corticosteroid medication for all young patients who have congestive heart failure which is not secondary to valvular or coronary heart diseases or to hypertrophic cardiomyopathy. Possibly, if the corticosteroid treatment had been continued for a longer period and with higher doses, improvement may have occurred.

Sudden death is one of the well recognized modes of death in patients with cardiac sarcoidosis.[1] Indeed, it is the most common mode of death in patients with cardiac sarcoidosis extensive enough to cause cardiac dysfunction, and it is the first manifestation of sarcoidosis in about 20 percent of patients with cardiac sarcoidosis. It is relatively unusual, however, for a patient with cardiac sarcoidosis and evidence of chronic congestive heart failure to die suddenly. Most patients with sudden death from cardiac sarcoidosis have preceding evidence of ventricular arrhythmias (most commonly ventricular tachycardia) or evidence of high degrees of heart block (most commonly complete heart block). Our patient never had evidence of multifocal or runs of ventricular premature beats or ventricular tachycardia or complete heart block.

One of the unique features of cardiac sarcoidosis is that patients with infiltration of the heart by sarcoid granulomas extensive enough to cause cardiac dysfunction infrequently have evidence of dysfunction of another body organ.[1] Our patient only had evidence of cardiac dysfunction and no dysfunction of another body organ. At necropsy, only sites where sarcoid granulomas were observed were in the heart, mediastinal lymph nodes, and lung

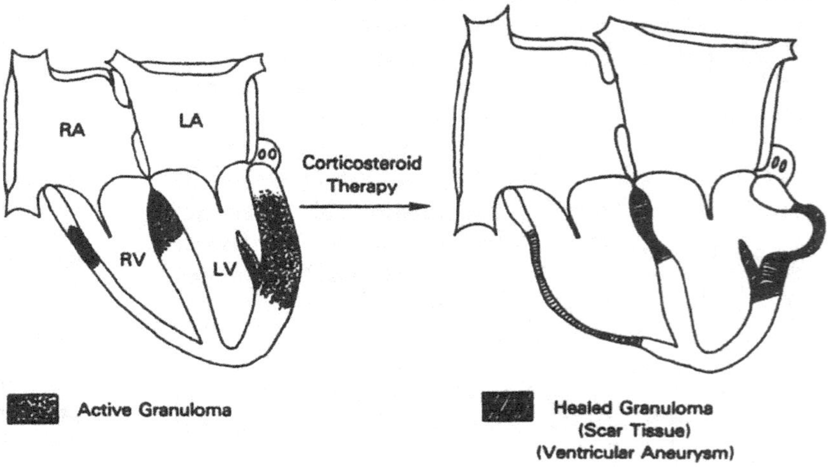

FIGURE 8. Good and bad effects of corticosteroid therapy in patients with cardiac sarcoidosis (reprinted with permission from Roberts WC, and the Yorke Medical Group[1]).

(one minute focus). A corollary to this is that the occurrence of symptomatic involvement of a noncardiac organ by sarcoid generally indicates that symptom-producing cardiac involvement by sarcoid is unlikely to occur. Flemming,[2] in search of patients with cardiac sarcoid, surveyed the chest, eye, and skin clinics in his hospital for patients with sarcoidosis and found this search unprofitable in revealing patients with cardiac sarcoid. Thus, cardiac sarcoidosis severe enough to cause cardiac dysfunction tends to be an all-or-none process: if it causes cardiac dysfunction, it tends not to cause dysfunction of another organ system; conversely, if it causes dysfunction of a noncardiac organ, it infrequently causes cardiac dysfunction. Although patients with fatal cardiac sarcoidosis may have sarcoid granulomas in other body organs, the extent of the sarcoid granulomas in the heart, in general, appears to be out of proportion to the extent in other body organs. Our patient had extensive granulomatous infiltrates in his myocardium, particularly the ventricles, but only one sarcoid granuloma was found in the lung and the only other body organ containing granuloma was lymph node.

One of the unusual histologic findings in sections of myocardium in our patient were granulomas around intramural coronary arteries. Dr. Virmani, can you summarize observations of others regarding cardiac sarcoid granulomas and their relationship to the coronary arteries?

Dr. Virmani: No one has reported sarcoid granulomas in extramural coronary arteries, but Morales and associates,[3] and more recently, James[4] pointed out that granulomas frequently surround the intramural coronary arteries of either cardiac atria or ventricles or both, and that the lumens of these arteries may be narrowed. The narrowing, in general, appears to result from intimal proliferation rather than from actual granulomatous invasion of the lumens. The medial and adventitial walls, however, have been observed to contain sarcoid granulomas. In our patient granulomas surrounded many intramural coronary arteries, particularly in the ventricles, and epithelioid cells were found to invade the wall of several intramural coronary arteries. Thus, sarcoidosis must be added to the list of causes of intramural coronary arterial disease. The functional significance of the involvement of the intramural coronary arteries, however, is uncertain. We suspect that it has little to no functional significance. Involvement of the small arteries in the lung by sarcoid granuloma has been noted in the past by others.[5] There is no surprise, therefore, that the small cardiac arteries may be involved by sarcoid granulomas.

Dr. Roberts: Dr. Virmani, the diagnosis of cardiac sarcoidosis clinically generally appears to be either simple or extremely difficult. Is this diagnosis easy at necropsy, and what morphologic criteria should be used to establish the diagnosis of cardiac sarcoidosis?

Dr. Virmani: To make the diagnosis of cardiac sarcoidosis at necropsy, we have required the presence of noncaseating granulomas in heart muscle and in lymph nodes.[1] The absence of noncaseating granulomas in lymph nodes, but their presence in the heart does not allow one to say, in our view, that sarcoidosis is the proper diagnosis. There have been a number of patients described with so-called "giant cell myocarditis." We believe that most of these patients in actuality had cardiac sarcoidosis. A problem here is that sarcoid may extensively involve the heart, and yet, although granulomas may be present in lymph nodes, the lymph nodes may not be enlarged. Because they are not enlarged at autopsy, histologic sections may not be prepared from them. If histologic sections are not prepared, certainly one cannot confirm or deny the presence of granulomas in these structures.

Dr. Roberts: One final comment regarding treatment. It seems reasonable to treat with corticosteroids any patient with documented cardiac sarcoidosis, be he (she) symptomatic or asymptomatic. As shown in the accompanying diagram (Fig 8), it appears that corticosteroid therapy causes shrinkage and conversion of the sarcoid granulomas into relatively dense scar tissue. In our patient, the cardiac sarcoid granulomas appeared quite active in that numerous lymphocytes surrounded the epithelioid and giant cell granulomas. In patients treated for long periods with corticosteroids, the cardiac sarcoid granulomas tend to be converted to scar tissue and the granulomas may disappear entirely. In our patient, relatively little myocardial scarring was observed.

References

1 Roberts WC, McAllister HA Jr, Ferrans VJ: Sarcoidosis of the heart; a clinicopathologic study of 35 necropsy patients (Group I) and review of 78 previously described necropsy patients (Group II). Am J Med 1977; 63:86

2 Flemming HA: Sarcoid heart disease. Br Med J 1973; 1:174

3 Morales AR, Levy S, Davis J, Fine G: Sarcoidosis and the heart. Pathol Ann 1974; 9:139

4 James TN: Sarcoid heart disease. Circulation 1977; 56:320

5 Carrington CB, Gaensler EA, Mikus JP, Schachter AW, Burke GW, Goff AM: Structure and function of sarcoidosis. Ann NY Acad Sci 1976; 278-265

Pulmonary Sarcoidosis: A Disease Characterized and Perpetuated by Activated Lung T-Lymphocytes

Moderator: RONALD G. CRYSTAL, M.D. *Discussants:* WILLIAM C. ROBERTS, M.D.; GARY W. HUNNINGHAKE, M.D.; JAMES E. GADEK, M.D.; JACK D. FULMER, M.D.; and BRUCE R. LINE, M.D.; Bethesda, Maryland

The alveolitis of pulmonary sarcoidosis is characterized by an intense, mononuclear cell infiltrate that probably precedes granuloma formation. Pathogenic mechanisms underlying pulmonary sarcoidosis can be shown by study of the mononuclear cells composing the alveolitis. Bronchoalveolar lavage has shown that the sarcoid lung is characterized by increased numbers of "activated" T-lymphocytes within the alveolar structures. In contrast to normal control cells, the lung T-lymphocytes of patients with sarcoid release the mediator, monocyte chemotactic factor, that probably contributes to the pathogenesis of sarcoidosis by recruiting blood monocytes to the lung, thus providing cellular building blocks for granuloma formation. Conventional monitors of the activity of pulmonary sarcoidosis, such as blood studies, pulmonary function testing, and chest roentgenograms, show little relation to the intensity of the T-lymphocyte alveolitis as assessed by bronchoalveolar lavage or by histopathologic studies. In contrast, quantification of lavage T-lymphocyte populations and ^{67}Ga scintigraphy of the chest provide a sensitive and specific means of assessing the activity of the alveolitis in pulmonary sarcoidosis and may provide a rational basis for therapy.

DR. RONALD G. CRYSTAL (Chief, Pulmonary Branch, National Heart, Lung, and Blood Institute): Sarcoidosis is a multisystem disease of undetermined cause characterized by the presence of noncaseating granulomas in many organs (1-6). Although the cause is unknown and the morphologic findings nonspecific, the combination of clinical, roentgenographic, histologic, and physiologic findings are so characteristic that in modern clinical practice the diagnosis of sarcoidosis is usually unambiguous (6-11). Sarcoidosis has been described in most tissues of the body, but for most patients lung involvement has the most serious consequences. At least 90% of all patients have pulmonary manifestations (1, 3-6, 12-14). Of these, 20% to 25% will have permanent loss of lung function, and 5% to 10% will die from the disease (1, 3, 4, 14-18).

The presence of granulomas in the alveolar structures in pulmonary sarcoidosis has long been considered histologic evidence that there are heightened cellular immune processes. However, many studies have documented a nonspecific depression of cellular immunity in this disorder. For example, most patients with active sarcoidosis have anergy to skin tests (12, 19, 20), impairment of the in-vitro proliferative response of blood mononuclear cells to antigens and mitogens (21-23), and a peripheral blood T-lymphocytopenia (24-28).

One explanation for this apparent paradox is that studies of uninvolved tissues such as skin and blood do not reflect the ongoing immune processes at the site of granuloma formation. The development of methods to directly evaluate the inflammatory and immune effector systems within the human lung has led to remarkable insights into the pathogenesis of this disease. Specifically, by 1978 it had become obvious that pulmonary sarcoidosis is characterized and perpetuated by increased numbers of activated T-lymphocytes within the alveolar structures (28-34).

To show the importance and ramifications of lung T-lymphocytes in this disease, we have used a study population of 45 persons with biopsy proven pulmonary sarcoidosis. Included were 20 males and 25 females, with an average age of 37 $\pm$ 5 years (all data are presented as the mean $\pm$ SE). By conventional clinical criteria, 19 were classified as having "active" disease.

First, we will define the disease morphologically, stressing the temporal sequence of the histologic findings. Second, we will detail the types, numbers, and function of lung inflammatory and immune effector cells, emphasizing the critical role of lung T-lymphocytes. Third, we will evaluate the tests available for staging sarcoidosis in terms of the sensitivity and specificity of these methods in staging the activity of the disease within the alveolar structures. Finally, we will review the therapy of pulmonary sarcoidosis, emphasizing the importance of using measures of inflammatory and immune activity within the lung as criteria for making decisions.

Morphologic Aspects

Dr. William C. Roberts (Chief, Pathology Branch, National Heart, Lung, and Blood Institute): The characteristic morphologic feature of pulmonary sarcoidosis is the presence of multiple noncaseating granulomas in the lung (Figure 1, *upper left*). The granulomas are always present in the alveolar septa (Figure 1, *upper right*) and usually in the walls of bronchi, pulmonary arteries, and veins (Figure 1, *lower left* and *right*) (1-3, 7, 35, 36).

COMPOSITION OF THE SARCOID GRANULOMA

The sarcoid granuloma is usually sharply circumscribed. Its central follicle consists of tightly packed cells,

▶ An edited transcription of a Combined Clinical Staff Conference at the Clinical Center, Bethesda, Maryland, 29 June 1978, by the National Institutes of Health, U.S. Department of Health, Education, and Welfare.

▶ Authors who wish to cite a section of the conference and specifically indicate its author can use this example for the form of reference:
ROBERTS WC. Morphologic aspects of pulmonary sarcoidosis, pp. 73-6. In: CRYSTAL RG, moderator. Pulmonary sarcoidosis: a disease characterized and perpetuated by activated lung T-lymphocytes. *Ann Intern Med.* 1981;94:73-94.

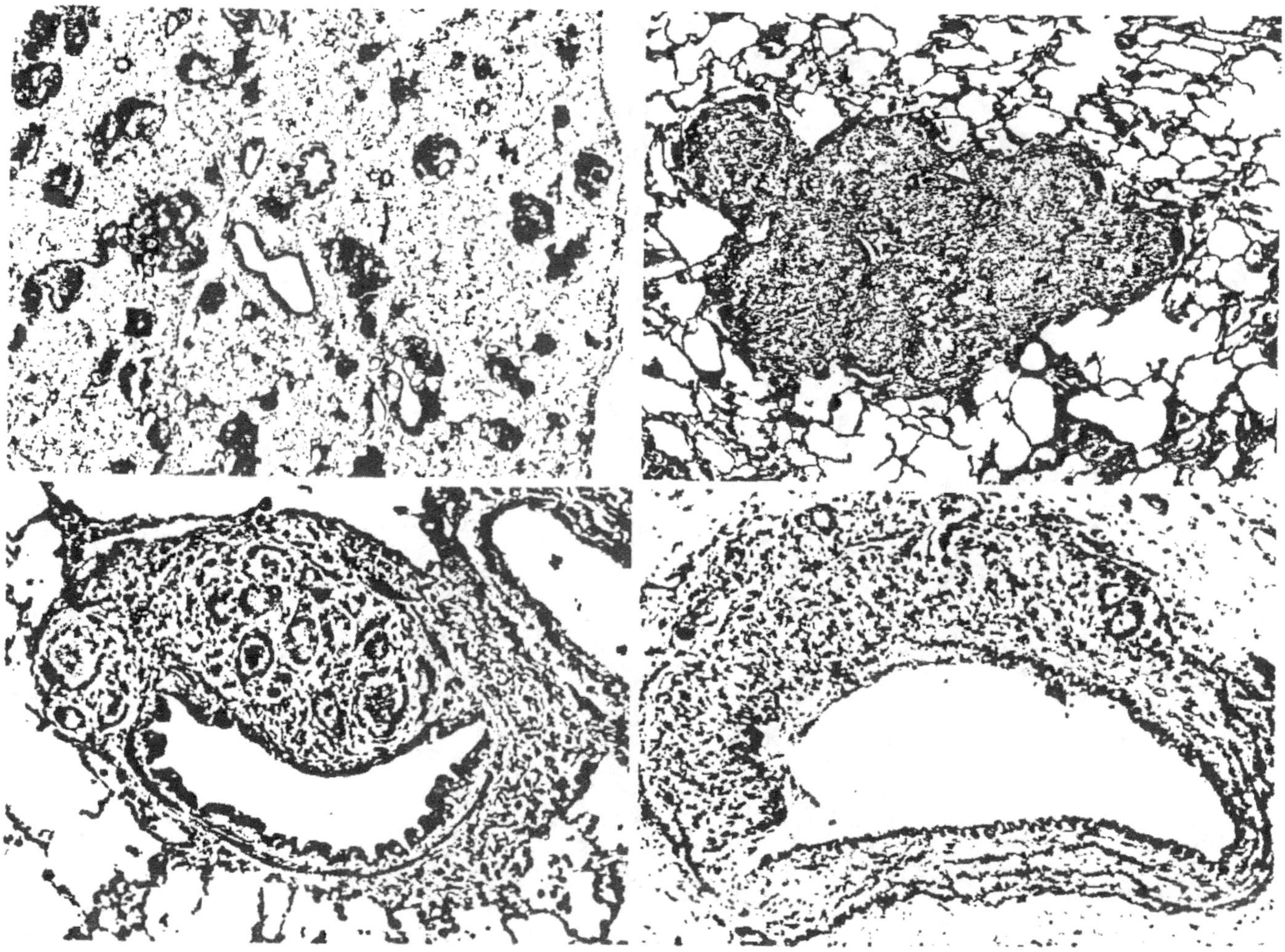

Figure 1. Pulmonary sarcoidosis. **Upper Left.** Multiple sarcoid granulomas with relative sparing of the pulmonary parenchyma between the granulomas. (Movat stain; original magnification, × 10.) **Upper Right.** A single large sarcoid granuloma with many mononuclear cells in the periphery. (Hematoxylin and eosin; original magnification, × 35.) **Lower Left.** The lumen of a bronchiole is compressed by a sarcoid granuloma. (Hematoxylin and eosin; original magnification, × 130.) **Lower Right.** A large pulmonary artery with a sarcoid granuloma in its wall ("sarcoid arteritis"). (Movat stain; original magnification, × 130.)

the major one being the so-called epithelioid cell. Surrounding the central follicle is a perimeter of lymphocytes, macrophages, monocytes, and fibroblasts (37, 38). The sarcoid granuloma is similar in appearance to those in all other types of granulomatous disease with the exception of tuberculosis (1-6).

Epithelioid cells occupy the body of the follicle as nodular collections of tightly packed cells. The term *epithelioid* was originally used because the size and arrangement of the cells were similar to the cells of epithelium; the epithelioid cell is now known, however, to be derived from the mononuclear-phagocyte system (39). Because epithelioid cells do have abundant cytoplasmic organelles, it has been suggested that they have secretory capabilities (40-42). Several populations of epithelioid cells have been described, but these "subclasses" are now believed to represent stages in the development of one cell type (6, 42-44).

Multinucleated giant cells, often up to 150 μm in diameter, are frequently found among the epithelioid cells within the granuloma follicle. The giant cells most commonly are of the Langhans' type with multiple, peripherally located, irregular nuclei (2, 3, 42). The cytoplasmic and nuclear features are identical to those of epithelioid cells (37).

The macrophages within the follicle are 10 to 25 μm in diameter and have numerous cytoplasmic processes that interdigitate with those of adjacent cells. The nuclei are indented and contain finely dispersed chromatin. The macrophages are rich in cytoplasmic organelles; but like epithelioid cells, the macrophages have a paucity of phagosomes or phagolysosomes, suggesting that they are not actively involved in phagocytosis (37). However, the macrophages within the granulomas do have numerous electron-dense lysosomes, suggesting that they are secretory cells (45).

The monocytes of the sarcoid follicle have a smoother surface then the macrophages (37). The nuclei are dark, and the cytoplasm has fewer organelles then the macrophage or epithelioid cell. Many of the lymphocytes of the follicle have the morphologic features of *activated* lymphocytes (37, 42, 43, 46). They are larger than the usual

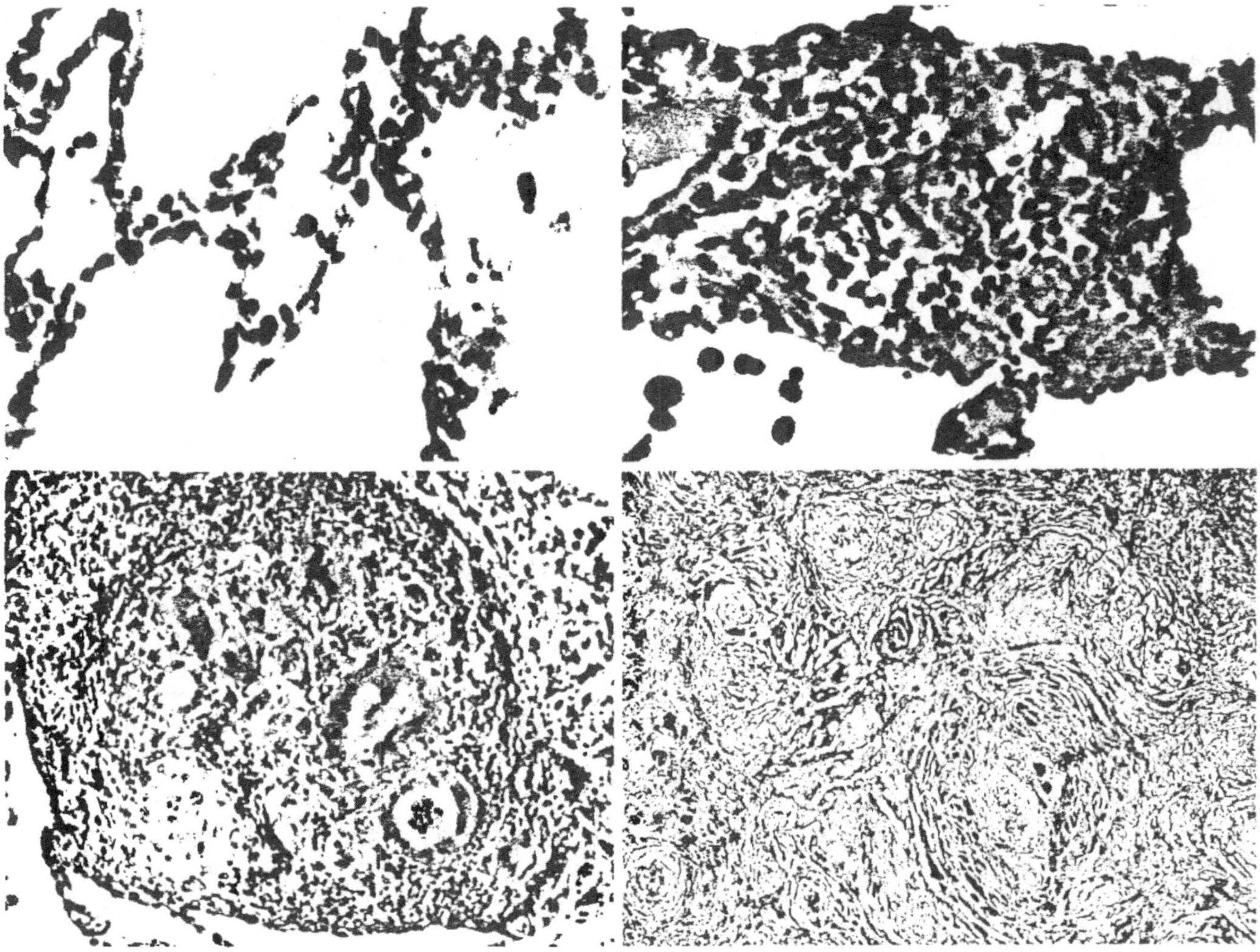

Figure 2. Stages of pulmonary sarcoidosis. **Upper Left.** Alveolar septae with increased numbers of mononuclear cells ("sarcoid alveolitis") Hematoxylin and eosin; original magnification, × 500.) **Upper Right.** Larger collection of mononuclear cells with few epithelioid cells and one giant cell in an alveolar septum. (Hematoxylin and eosin; original magnification, × 500.) **Lower Left.** A well-developed sarcoid granuloma with many giant cells and mononuclear cells only in the periphery. (Hematoxylin and eosin; original magnification, × 220.) **Lower Right.** The final stage in the organization of a sarcoid granuloma. The granulomas now consist mainly of relatively dense fibrous tissue, and only an occasional giant or epithelioid cell remains. (Hematoxylin and eosin; original magnification, × 55.)

lymphocyte and contain an irregular nucleus, often with centrioles; the cytoplasm contains large numbers of mitochrondria, dense granules, ribosomes, and rough endoplasmic reticulum.

The extracellular material within and surrounding the central follicle is classically described as *amorphous hyaline material* or *reticulin* (2). Although it has been suggested that some of this material was "para-amyloid" (47), electron microscopy has shown that it is mostly ground substance with interspersed fibers of various diameters (48). The exact nature of the latter is unknown. It has been described as amyloid or fibrin-like, but is more likely one or more types of collagen.

When involving alveolar septa, the sarcoid granuloma distorts the interstitium by its physical bulk and, thus, probably causes derangements in air-blood relations (37, 49). The presence of granulomas, however, does not seem to affect structures composing the so-called alveolar-capillary membrane; measurements of the pathway between air and blood in the sarcoid lung have shown it to be normal or, at most, slightly increased (50).

ALVEOLITIS OF SARCOIDOSIS; EVOLUTION OF DISEASE

Whereas early reports described the granuloma of sarcoid as being monotonously uniform (suggesting they begin at the same time) (51), it is now clear that the lesions of pulmonary sarcoidosis can originate at different times (5, 6). Moreover, although the granulomas are the morphologic hallmarks of pulmonary sarcoidosis, the alveolar structures in this disease also are characterized by accumulations of inflammatory and immune-effector cells within the interstitium and alveolus (5, 36, 52). Commonly referred to as the *alveolitis* of sarcoidosis, these inflammatory and immune effector cell accumulations consist of monocytes, macrophages, and lymphocytes that are present in approximately equal numbers. In most patients, the majority of effector cells are found within the interstitium rather than the alveolar air spaces (36, 52).

Although the diagnosis of sarcoidosis cannot be made without the presence of granulomas, there is increasing evidence that the alveolitis of sarcoidosis precedes the formation of the granulomas (Figure 2) (34, 36, 52-55). The extensive studies by Rosen and associates (52) have shown that early, developing granulomas are composed of a loose collection of inflammatory and immune effector cells in which monocytes, macrophages, and lymphocytes predominate over epithelioid cells. As the granuloma matures, numbers of epithelioid cells increase and numbers of monocytes, macrophages, and lymphocytes decrease (37, 52, 56). In patients with extensive alveolitis, few granulomas are present, but in patients with numerous granulomas, the alveolitis is minimal or absent, further supporting the concept that the alveolitis precedes the granulomas (52). At least part of the alveolitis of sarcoidosis is derived from circulating inflammatory and immune effector cells; Soler and Bassett (37) have presented morphologic evidence that blood monocytes pass from capillaries to the interstitium in this disease.

The fate of the sarcoid granuloma has been well documented morphologically. Although it can appear *fresh* from months to years, the granuloma ultimately either resolves leaving few or no morphologic changes or it undergoes progressive fibrosis (1, 5, 6, 57). The fibrosis begins as a rim of collagen around the granuloma and proceeds in a centripetal fashion until the entire structure is replaced by fibrous tissue (1, 2, 37, 53, 56). It is likely, although unproven, that the collagen composing the fibrous tissue originates from the fibroblasts in the periphery of the granuloma (37). As the lesion "matures," fibroblasts proliferate in the periphery of the granuloma (56). In older granulomas, peripheral fibroblasts are extensive, and the inflammatory and immune effector cells in the periphery of the granuloma disappear (56). As the fibrosis proceeds inward, capillaries in the region are trapped and disappear (37, 55).

In about 20% of patients with sarcoidosis, there is progression to interstitial fibrosis, distortion, and replacement of the pulmonary architecture (58, 59). These progressive lesions are associated with increased amounts of collagen fibers within the interstitium, obliteration of capillaries, and destruction of architecture by inflammatory and immune effector cells, granulomas, and fibroblasts (37). Eventually, the normal alveolar architecture disappears, resulting in cystic spaces interspersed with bands of connective tissue producing the so-called *end-stage*.

Thus, on morphologic grounds, pulmonary sarcoidosis appears to begin as a mononuclear alveolitis that proceeds to a multinucleated, giant cell granulomatous disease. Thereafter, two alternatives are available: The granulomas resolve leaving relatively normal lung (80% of patients), or progressive fibrosis ensues producing end-stage lung. In either case, the process takes place in various alveolar structures at different times and progresses at different rates.

Characterization of the Alveolitis of Sarcoidosis

Dr. Gary W. Hunninghake (Senior Investigator, Pulmonary Branch, National Heart, Lung, and Blood Institute): Pulmonary sarcoidosis is characterized by the presence of granulomas in the lung parenchyma (5, 6, 60). However, as we have just seen, the earliest lesion of this disease is an alveolitis, a diffuse infiltration of the lung parenchyma by mononuclear cells (36, 52-54). We may conceive, therefore, of the sequence of events in the development of pulmonary sarcoidosis as follows. A stimulus, at present not defined, results in an accumulation of mononuclear cells in the lung parenchyma (that is, the alveolitis). The alveolitis either resolves spontaneously or leads to the formation of granulomas. The presence of granulomas is usually associated with at least some degree of alteration of interstitial connective tissue and epithelial, endothelial, and mesenchymal cells that compose the normal alveolar structures. Although whether it is the alveolitis or granulomas, or both, that mediate these alterations is unclear, it is evident that in some cases the derangement of the alveolar structure is progressive, leading to interstitial fibrosis and the eventual end-stage of alveolar-capillary units.

The sequence of events outlined above does not take place in all of the alveolar structures at the same time or at the same rate. Rather, small groups of units are affected at different times and progress through the phases of alveolitis to granulomas, fibrosis, and cellular derangement to end-stage at different rates. Also, the disease within each group of alveoli may halt, resolve, or progress, making the overall picture a montage of alveolar-capillary units in various stages of inflammation and derangement. Thus, a patient with sarcoidosis will have some alveoli that are normal, some with alveolitis, and others with various mixtures of alveolitis, granuloma, fibrosis, and alterations of parenchymal cells. Over a time, the number of units in each phase will probably change, giving an overall picture of either no lung disease, stable lung disease, or progressive lung disease.

On the basis of these observations, it is clear that characterization and quantification of the alveolitis of sarcoidosis is an important means of defining the pathogenesis as well as the activity and prognosis of the disease.

TECHNIQUE

The inflammatory and immune effector cells forming the alveolitis of sarcoidosis can be recovered from the alveolar structures by a technique termed *bronchoalveolar lavage* (28, 32-34, 61-64). With this method, the effector cells within the lower respiratory tract are obtained by placing a fiberoptic bronchoscope in a distal airway, instilling 1 dL of sterile saline in five 20-mL aliquots, and recovering the lavage fluid by suction. With this technique, from 10 to 30 $\times$ 10^6 effector cells can be recovered; with the immunologic methods now available, this is sufficient to permit detailed characterization of the type, number, and state of activation of the cells that are present. Also, because bronchoalveolar lavage is rapid and safe, the procedure can be used to contrast the effector cell populations of the lungs of sarcoidosis patients with those of normal persons and of persons with other lung disorders and can be used to evaluate the effector cell populations of the same patient over a period of time.

One area of concern in using bronchoalveolar lavage to evaluate the inflammatory and immune effector cell populations in the lower respiratory tract is the possibility that the cells recovered by lavage do not accurately reflect the true alveolitis of the disease. However, studies comparing the effector cells in open lung biopsies of patients to the effector cells recovered by lavage have shown that the cells recovered by lavage accurately reflect the ongoing inflammatory and immune processes within the lower respiratory tract (31, 33, 65). In addition, the inflammatory and immune effector cells obtained by lavage of one segment of the lung appear to be representative of the alveolitis of the sarcoid lung as a whole (66). Although it is not known how many alveolar-capillary units are washed out during the lavage procedure, it is apparent that enough alveoli are sampled so that the local differences from one group of alveolar-capillary units to another are averaged out in the lavage specimen.

The current methods of handling the lavage fluid and characterizing and quantifying the recovered cells have been detailed in a recent review (33). The cell populations are usually quantified as a percentage of the total bronchoalveolar cells. Quantifying the absolute numbers of these cells is not very meaningful, because the yield of cells may be influenced by multiple factors such as the placement of the bronchoscope or the relative "stickiness" of the cells to the alveolar epithelial surface.

GENERAL CHARACTERISTICS OF THE ALVEOLITIS OF SARCOIDOSIS

Evaluation of the inflammatory and immune effector cell populations recovered from the lungs of patients with sarcoidosis shows that the alveolitis of this disease contrasts sharply with the effector cell populations of normal lung and is markedly different than the alveolitis of most other interstitial disorders (28, 32-34, 63-71).

The effector cells present in the alveolar structures of normal nonsmokers consist of more than 90% alveolar macrophages, less than 10% lymphocytes, and less than 1% polymorphonuclear leukocytes (28, 32, 33, 64). In contrast, sarcoidosis is characterized by a marked increase in the proportions of lymphocytes in the lower respiratory tract (28, 31-34, 63-71). On the average, our study population had 33% ± 6% lymphocytes in their lavage fluid compared to less than 10% for normal nonsmokers and smokers. In our sarcoidosis patients with clinical criteria associated with active disease (such as fever, weight loss, erythema nodosum, progressive deterioration of lung function) the proportion of lung lymphocytes was 55% ± 8%, almost twofold higher than that of the group average.

Most other interstitial disorders are associated with normal proportions of lymphocytes in the alveolar structures. Other than sarcoidosis, the only lung disorders know to be associated with increased proportions of lymphocytes in lavage fluid are hypersensitivity pneumonitis (62), tuberculosis (33, 72), and lymphoma involving the lung parenchyma (33). As more lung disorders are evaluated by bronchoalveolar lavage, this list is likely to grow; from the pattern emerging, it will probably include most granulomatous lung diseases in addition to lymphocyte-derived malignancies involving lung parenchyma (33).

In addition to lymphocytes, the remainder of the effector cells characterizing the alveolitis of sarcoidosis are monocytes and macrophages (5, 6, 28, 31-34, 36, 52-54, 61-71); as in normal persons, nonsmoking patients with sarcoidosis have less than 1% neutrophils in their lower respiratory tract (28-34, 64, 65). With the technology presently available, it is not possible to distinguish between the small young macrophage and the blood monocyte that has recently migrated to the alveolar structures; hence the terms *macrophages* or *mononuclear phagocytes* are used interchangeably when this population of cells in bronchoalveolar lavage fluid analyses is discussed. Although the proportions of these cells are lower in lavage fluid recovered from patients with sarcoidosis as compared to those in normal persons, it is important to emphasize that the total number of inflammatory and immune effector cells in the sarcoid lung is many times that in the normal lung. Thus, in terms of total numbers, the alveolitis of sarcoidosis is characterized not only by increased numbers of lymphocytes but also by increased numbers of mononuclear phagocytes.

From these studies, it is apparent that bronchoalveolar lavage analysis yields a picture of the alveolitis of pulmonary sarcoidosis similar to that of the open lung biopsy: Sarcoidosis is a disease characterized by the accumulation of large numbers of lymphocytes, monocytes, and macrophages within the alveolar structures.

CHARACTERIZATION AND QUANTIFICATION OF LYMPHOCYTE SUBTYPES

Estimates of the relative numbers of lymphocyte subtypes in the lower respiratory tract can be expressed either as a percentage of the total lymphocytes present or as a percentage of total inflammatory and immune effector cells present. Both methods are valuable, as they give somewhat different insights into the importance of the various cells as components of the inflammatory and immune effector cell populations of the lower respiratory tract. Whereas expressing the numbers of lymphocyte subtypes as a percentage of total lymphocytes present gives an estimate of relative shifts in lymphocyte subpopulations, expressing the numbers of lymphocyte subtypes as a percentage of total alveolar effector cells gives an estimate of the overall intensity of each lymphocyte component of the pulmonary inflammatory and immune process.

In normal persons, the percentage of lung lymphocytes that is T-lymphocytes varies from 65% to 80%; this is also the case for interstitial disorders such as idiopathic pulmonary fibrosis, the collagen-vascular disorders, and histiocytosis-X (28, 32, 33, 64). In marked contrast, our study population with sarcoidosis, unselected for disease activity, had an average of 90% ± 4% of all lung lymphocytes as T-lymphocytes. In fact, T-lymphocytes represented more than 80% (the high normal value) of all lung lymphocytes in 91% of the persons in the study population, in spite of the fact that these patients were unselected in terms of any clinical, roentgenographic, or physiologic criteria. Of the patients with less than 80% T-lymphocytes, none had any evidence of lung disease at

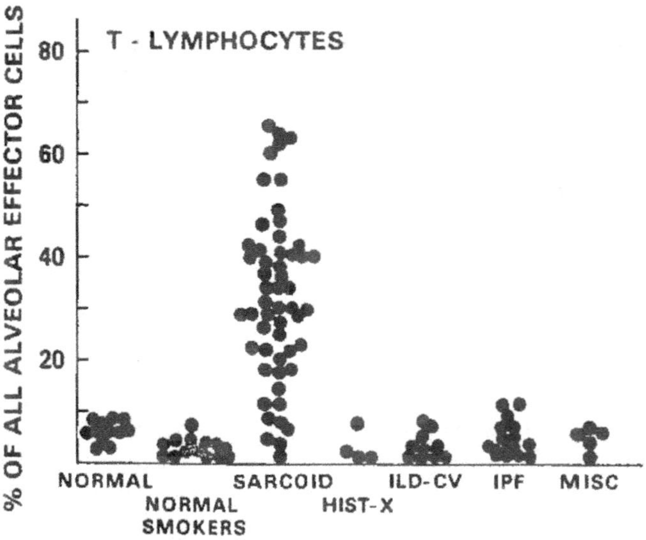

Figure 3. Proportion of all inflammatory and immune effector cells in the alveolar structures that are T-lymphocytes in normal persons and in persons with various chronic lung disorders, including untreated patients with sarcoidosis. The lung effector cells were recovered by bronchoalveolar lavage. For normal persons (nonsmokers and smokers), T-lymphocytes represent less than 8% of all effector cells present. Hist-X = histiocytosis-X; ILD-CV = interstitial lung disease associated with collagen vascular disease (included are patients with rheumatoid arthritis, progressive systemic sclerosis, systemic lupus erythematosus, and mixed connective tissue disease); IPF = idiopathic pulmonary fibrosis; Misc = various miscellaneous lung disorders (included are patients with familial pulmonary fibrosis, Kartagener's syndrome, inorganic dust disease, squamous cell carcinoma, and cystic fibrosis).

the time of evaluation. Thus, pulmonary sarcoidosis is a disease characterized by shifts in the proportions of lung lymphocytes toward more T-lymphocytes (28-34, 65).

That patients with pulmonary sarcoidosis have increased proportions of T-lymphocytes in their alveolar structures is even more remarkable when compared to the findings in their peripheral blood. Although these persons have large amounts of T-lymphocytes in lung, they simultaneously have peripheral blood T-lymphocytopenia (23-34), suggesting that observations of cellular immune processes in blood may give a false view of what is actually occurring in lung. In comparison to persons with sarcoidosis, normal persons have the same proportions of T-lymphocytes in lung and blood as do patients with idiopathic pulmonary fibrosis, interstitial lung disease associated with collagen-vascular disease, and histiocytosis-X (28, 32, 33).

When the numbers of T-lymphocytes in the sarcoid lung are expressed as a proportion of the total inflammatory and immune effector cells present, it becomes apparent that this disease is characterized not only by shifts in the proportions of lung lymphocytes that are T-lymphocytes but also by an intense T-lymphocyte alveolitis. Whereas in normal persons, T-lymphocytes account for less than 8% of all inflammatory and immune effector cells within the alveolar structures, in persons with sarcoidosis, T-lymphocytes represent 31% ± 8% of the effector cells present (Figure 3). By comparison, in most other interstitial disorders, less than 8% of all effector cells present in the lower respiratory tract are T-lymphocytes (28-33). This increased proportion of T-lymphocytes in the sarcoid lung becomes even more impressive when one considers that although normal persons have approximately 25×10^9 effector cells in their lower respiratory tract (73), morphologic observations of biopsies of patients with sarcoidosis with active alveolitis suggest that there are probably five to 20 times more effector cells within their alveolar structures (5, 6, 36, 52-54, 60). It is apparent, therefore, that in absolute numbers T-lymphocytes are tremendously increased within the alveolar structures of the sarcoid lung.

Although the proportions of lung lymphocytes that are T-lymphocytes are increased in the sarcoid lung, the proportions of lung lymphocytes that are B-lymphocytes are significantly reduced (28, 32, 33). In contrast, the proportions of lymphocytes that are B-lymphocytes are increased in the blood of sarcoid patients compared to their own lungs and to the blood of normal persons. Because the sarcoid lung is characterized by an overall increase in total lymphocytes, it is likely that the total number of B-lymphocytes is increased within the sarcoid lung even though the proportion of these cells is reduced. Even so, the total number of T-lymphocytes is still far in excess; on the average, the sarcoid lung has 20 to 25 times more T-lymphocytes than B-lymphocytes (28-33). In comparison, the normal lung has only seven to 10 times more T-lymphocytes than B-lymphocytes (28-33).

If, as suggested above, lung T-lymphocytes are actively involved in the pathogenesis of pulmonary sarcoidosis, many of these lung T-lymphocytes are probably in a state of relative activation and thus function as effector T-lymphocytes. In support of this concept are the findings that in parallel with the marked increase in the numbers of T-lymphocytes in the sarcoid lung, there are also increases in numbers of various subtypes of T-lymphocytes in the alveolar structures of these patients (28-34). Most importantly, persons with sarcoidosis have increased proportions of lung T-lymphocytes that form rosettes with sheep erythrocytes at 37 °C, a subset of T-lymphocytes well known to be in a relative state of activation (Figure 4) (28, 32, 33, 74, 75). Additional evidence of increased numbers of activated T-lymphocytes in the lungs of sarcoid patients comes from the observation that these patients have increased numbers of T-lymphocytes that have receptors for the crystallizable fragment (Fc) portion of IgG (so-called $T\gamma$ cells) (28, 32, 33). Although the exact role of $T\gamma$ cells in the pathogenesis of sarcoidosis is unknown, several studies have shown that increased numbers of this subset of T-lymphocytes are present when a population of T-lymphocytes has been activated in some manner (76-78).

As pointed out by other investigators, there are increased proportions of T-lymphocytes forming rosettes with sheep erythrocytes at 37 °C (79) and $T\gamma$ cells (80) in the blood of patients with sarcoid compared to blood of normals. Although this was also true in our study population, the proportion and total numbers of these T-lymphocyte subtypes in blood were far less than those found in lung, further suggesting that analysis of blood does not give a true picture of the character and magnitude of the immune processes within the lung.

Further evidence of the presence of increased numbers of activated T-lymphocytes in the sarcoid lung comes from studies of the relative proportions of these cells undergoing spontaneous transformation. In this regard, unstimulated, highly purified T-lymphocytes isolated from the lungs of patients with sarcoidosis spontaneously incorporate three- to fourfold greater amounts of [^{3}H]thymidine than do equal numbers of lung T-lymphocytes from normal persons (HUNNINGHAKE GW, CRYSTAL RG. Unpublished observations). In addition, as will be discussed by Dr. Gadek, lung T-lymphocytes from patients with sarcoidosis spontaneously release a variety of lymphokines whereas lung T-lymphocytes from normal persons do not (28, 33, 34).

Thus, it is clear that the alveolitis of sarcoidosis is characterized by increased numbers of lymphocytes, monocytes, and macrophages. Whereas the effector role of the monocytes and macrophages in the sarcoid lung has not been evaluated, it is apparent that this disease is distinguished by large numbers of activated T-lymphocytes within the alveolar structures. Furthermore, these activated T-lymphocytes probably play a major role in the pathogenesis of the disease. Because the activity of the alveolitis can be accurately gauged by analysis of the cell populations in bronchoalveolar lavage fluid, this technique should prove useful in staging patients with sarcoidosis and following their response to therapy.

Maintenance of the Alveolitis of Sarcoidosis

Dr. James E. Gadek (Senior Investigator, Pulmonary Branch, National Heart, Lung, and Blood Institute): Although the initiating stimulus for sarcoidosis is unknown, increasingly there are clues as to how the sarcoid granuloma is formed and maintained. As discussed by Drs. Roberts and Hunninghake, the appearance of granuloma is preceded by an accumulation of monocytes, macrophages, and lymphocytes, particularly T-lymphocytes, within the alveolar structures. I will outline the importance of all these cell types in forming and maintaining granuloma within the lower respiratory tract.

IMPORTANCE OF MONONUCLEAR PHAGOCYTES

Monocytes and alveolar macrophages are part of the *mononuclear phagocyte* system, a term applied to a specific class of phagocytic cells derived from monoblasts within the bone marrow (39, 81-83). The mononuclear phagocyte system forms a continuum of cells that progressively mature from precursor marrow cells to blood monocytes and finally to macrophages. In addition, the evidence is overwhelming that epithelioid cells and giant cells are derived from monocytes and macrophages (53, 54, 83-88). Thus, in pulmonary sarcoidosis, granuloma formation is conceived as a coalescence and maturation of mononuclear phagocytes that are in the alveolar structures. Consequently, although mononuclear phagocytes have a variety of effector functions that may be relevant to the pathogenesis of sarcoidosis (64, 68, 83, 89-98), one critical role of these cells in this disease is to serve as a building block for granuloma formation.

Because granulomas are dynamic structures, there is a need for the constant replenishment of mononuclear phagocytes as epithelioid cells and giant cells either die or move out of granuloma (85, 88). This constant requirement for a monocyte and macrophage pool in the formation of new granuloma and maintenance of established granuloma suggests processes that maintain the mononuclear phagocyte series of cells within the alveolar structures are relevant to the pathogenesis of sarcoidosis.

There are two mechanisms that could serve to replenish the monocyte and macrophage pool within the lung: Monocytes and macrophages within the alveolar structures could proliferate locally, or monocytes could be recruited to the lung from the blood monocyte pool, or both could occur. There are several reasons to think that the second mechanism is more important in pulmonary sarcoidosis. First, although monocytes and macrophages in the lower respiratory tract have the capacity to proliferate (99, 100), large numbers of monocytes and macrophages would have to be constantly dividing to maintain the monocyte series within the sarcoid lung (82). However, evaluation of biopsies of sarcoid lung rarely shows these cells in mitosis (2, 3, 36, 37). Second, studies with experimental models of granuloma formation have shown that most cells composing granuloma are derived from the circulating pool of blood monocytes (45, 53, 68, 83-88). Consistent with this concept, biopsies of patients with sarcoidosis show monocytes migrating from capillaries to the alveolar interstitium (37).

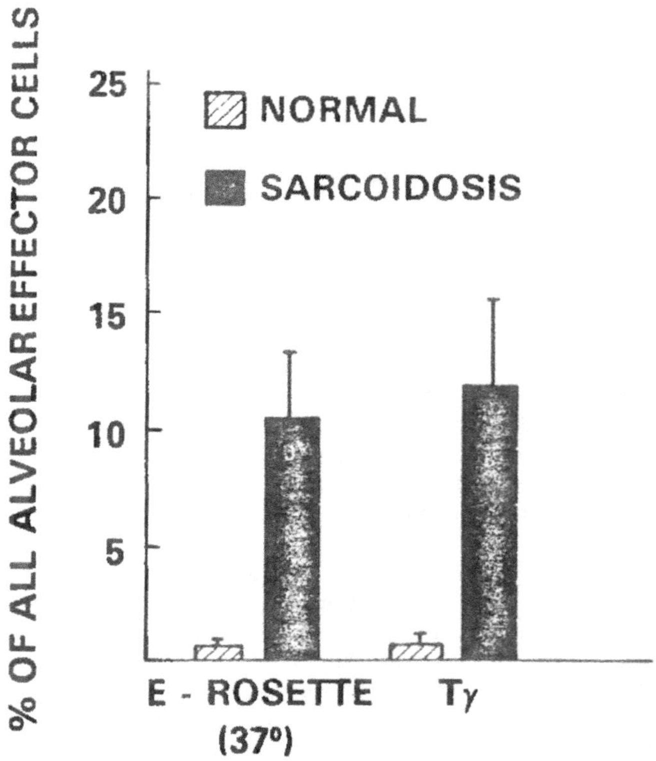

Figure 4. Subtypes of T-lymphocytes in the lungs of patients with sarcoidosis. Two subtypes of T-lymphocytes were evaluated, those forming rosettes with sheep erythrocytes at 37 °C (*E-Rosette, 37°*) and those with receptors for the Fc portion of IgG (*Tγ*). The data are presented as the proportions of all inflammatory and immune effector cells represented as each T-lymphocyte subtype. The normal study population consisted of eight persons and the sarcoid population, of nine. The error bars represent SEM.

Table 1. Role of Lung T-Lymphocytes in Recruiting Blood Monocytes to the Lung in Patients With Pulmonary Sarcoidosis*

Mediator	Function	Normal Persons†		Patients with Sarcoid†	
		Blood	Lung	Blood	Lung
Monocyte chemotactic factor‡	Recruitment of circulating monocytes to the site of mediator release	0	0	1+	4+
Leukocyte inhibitory factor§	Inhibition of polymorphonuclear leukocyte migration	0	0	1+	4+

* Production of soluble mediators of inflammatory cell migration by lung and blood T-lymphocytes of normal persons and patients with pulmonary sarcoidosis.
† Lung and blood T-lymphocytes were incubated for 48 h. at 37 °C and the supernatants evaluated for the production of monocyte chemotactic factor and leukocyte inhibitory factor. The relative amounts of the factors produced are expressed on an arbitrary scale of 0 (none) to 4+ (maximum, equivalent to mitogen-stimulated T-lymphocytes) (28, 34).
‡ Quantified using purified blood monocytes as target cells in a modified Boyden chemotaxis assay (34).
§ Quantified using unfractionated blood leukocytes as target cells in a chemotaxis under agarose assay (28).

MONOCYTE RECRUITMENT TO THE SARCOID LUNG: ROLE OF T-LYMPHOCYTES

The process of recruitment of leukocytes from one compartment to another is known as chemotaxis (101). Chemotactic stimuli are generally protein or lipid and are referred to as "chemotactic factors." A vast array of such factors has been described, some derived from serum and others produced directly by cells (102-115). In addition, a number of chemotactic inhibitors have been characterized (116-121), and thus the process of chemotaxis must be considered as a balance between the attractive nature of chemotactic factors and the restraining influence of chemotactic inhibitors. Whereas some of these processes are directed toward all leukocytes, others affect one cell type more than others allowing for the expression of specificity in cell migrations. This concept is important because neutrophils are rarely found in the sarcoid lung, suggesting that blood monocytes are recruited to the sarcoid lung, and blood neutrophils are excluded.

Chemotactic factors are conventionally evaluated in vitro by the use of chemotactic chambers in which the target cells and putative chemotactic stimuli are separated by a membrane of calibrated pore size. In such a system, chemotactic activity is usually quantitated as the number of target cells moving through the membrane toward the stimulus per unit time (122). To evaluate the role played by lung inflammatory and immune effector cells in recruiting blood monocytes, unstimulated lung T-lymphocytes obtained from sarcoid patients by bronchoalveolar lavage were cultured for 48 hours, after which the supernatants of these cells were evaluated for chemotactic activity using blood monocytes as target cells (34).

Such studies convincingly demonstrate that T-lymphocytes comprising the alveolitis of sarcoidosis are spontaneously elaborating a specific factor (monocyte chemotactic factor) that attracts blood monocytes (34) (Table 1). In contrast, T-lymphocytes present in normal alveolar structures have no influence on the migration of blood monocytes. Monocyte chemotactic factor has a molecular mass of 10 to 15 000 daltons and is probably a protein (110). Whereas T-lymphocytes from the normal lung can be induced to elaborate monocyte chemotactic factor (for example, by stimulation with a mitogen such as concanavalin A), the T-lymphocytes obtained from the lungs of sarcoid patients are spontaneously secreting it (34). This finding is consistent with the concept that increased numbers of T-lymphocytes found in the sarcoid lung are activated.

In addition, comparison of T-lymphocytes from lung and blood of sarcoid patients demonstrates that lung T-lymphocytes spontaneously secrete larger amounts of monocyte chemotactic factor than blood T-lymphocytes of the same person (Table 1). The difference between lung and blood is striking; sarcoid lung T-lymphocytes produce an average of 25 times more of this chemotactic factor per cell than do sarcoid blood T-lymphocytes (34). This observation, together with the finding that the sarcoid lung contains large numbers of T-lymphocytes, suggests that concentrations of this chemotactic factor are higher in lung than in blood. Thus, a gradient of monocyte chemotactic factor between lung and blood of these patients is likely, resulting in the chronic accumulation of blood monocytes within the alveolar structures. In light of this observation, it is not difficult to understand how the pool of mononuclear phagocytes may be maintained within the sarcoid lung, providing a continuous source of basic building blocks for granuloma formation.

Although the elaboration of monocyte chemotactic factor by sarcoid lung T-lymphocytes explains the attraction of blood monocytes to the lung in this disease, it does not explain why monocytes, and not polymorphonuclear leukocytes, are recruited. When neutrophils are used as the target cell, chemotactic chamber studies show that monocyte chemotactic factor attracts neutrophils as well as monocytes (123). Thus, we have to look elsewhere to explain the specificity of the recruitment of monocytes in this disease.

One clue comes from analysis of other products elaborated by activated T-lymphocytes. Along with monocyte chemotactic factor, lung T-lymphocytes from sarcoid patients also spontaneously produced leukocyte inhibitory factor (28), a 68 000-dalton product that prevents the migration of polymorphonuclear leukocytes, but not monocytes (119) (Table 1). In addition, patients with sarcoidosis have elevated levels of serum lysozyme (68), an enzyme that inhibits the migration of neutrophils (124). In sarcoidosis, therefore, blood leukocytes are probably under a number of attractive and inhibitory stimuli, the net result of which is to recruit monocytes, but no neutrophils, to the alveolar structures.

Various studies have shown that blood monocytes of sarcoid patients are in a relative state of activation compared to blood monocytes of normal persons. Monocytes of sarcoid patients have increased numbers of IgG-Fc and C3 receptors (125), show increased spreading (126), and contain more lysozyme (68, 127), β-galactosidase (128), and angiotensin-converting enzyme (68, 129-131), all of which are considered criteria for mononuclear phagocyte activation (68). Although the mechanism of monocyte activation in sarcoidosis is undoubtedly complex and involves a variety of processes, T-lymphocytes probably play a role. In this regard, products elaborated by activated T-lymphocytes are known to be able to stimulate blood monocytes as well as attract them (132). The results of monocyte activation are probably important in helping the monocyte negotiate tissue barriers in its migration from capillary lumen to alveolar interstitium and in preparing the monocyte for its role in granuloma formation. In addition, that lung T-lymphocytes from sarcoid patients also spontaneously elaborate macrophage migration inhibitory factor (HUNNINGHAKE GW, GADEK JE, CRYSTAL RG. Unpublished observations) may provide a mechanism for the immobilization of the monocyte once it arrives within the alveolar structures. Although the relative state of cells composing sarcoid granuloma has not yet been studied, evidence from other forms of granuloma, such as that found in tuberculosis and schistosomasis, suggests that monocytes, macrophages, and epithelioid cells forming granuloma are in a relative state of activation (68, 83-88).

In addition to locally produced T-lymphocyte products, numerous inhibitory factors have been found in serum of patients with sarcoidosis. Although these circulating inhibitory factors probably play an important role in the cutaneous anergy of sarcoidosis, their presence does not seem to be related to disease activity in the lung (133-141). Thus, their role, if any, in the recruitment of blood monocytes to the sarcoid lung is unclear.

In summary, quantitative analysis of the alveolitis of sarcoidosis has shown that it is made up of monocytes, macrophages, and lymphocytes, including large numbers of activated T-lymphocytes. Analysis of the products elaborated by T-lymphocytes composing the alveolitis of sarcoidosis shows that these cells produce factors whose net effect is to attract blood monocytes specifically. Although these observations are relevant only to a part of the pathogenesis of sarcoidosis, they explain how one important cellular constituent of the sarcoid alveolitis is maintained.

Skin Testing, Blood Studies, and Bronchoalveolar Lavage to Assess Activity

Dr. Ronald G. Crystal: Traditionally, the activity of pulmonary sarcoidosis has been assessed with a number of loosely defined clinical criteria such as the presence or absence of weight loss, fatigue, weakness, malaise, fever, erythema nodosum, dry cough, progressive dyspnea, and worsening exercise intolerance (1, 3-5, 7, 12-16, 35). However, true activity of pulmonary sarcoid can be defined only in terms of the actual disease process in the lung. Because the alveolitis of sarcoidosis clearly precedes, and probably causes, the anatomic derangements of the alveolar structures that are characteristic of this disease, assessments of disease activity must take into account the number, type, and functional state of the inflammatory and immune effector cells in the lower respiratory tract. Thus, in view of our previous discussions, monitors of disease activity should assess the status of lung T-lymphocytes, lung mononuclear phagocytes, or both.

Table 2. Skin Test and Blood Studies Suggested in the Literature as Means to Assess the Activity of Pulmonary Sarcoidosis

Test	References
Skin testing	
Evaluation of anergy to a variety of antigens	1, 3–5, 12, 19–23, 143–149
Rebuck skin window	170
Evaluation of circulating mononuclear cells	
Number of lymphocytes	24, 25, 146, 150–151
Number of T-lymphocytes	24–27, 145, 149, 151, 152
Number of activated T-lymphocytes	70, 79, 80, 153
Response of lymphocytes to mitogens and antigens	21–23, 35, 145, 146, 154, 155
Response of lymphocytes to mixed lymphocyte cultures	143
Generation of killer cells	143
Spontaneous production of migration inhibition factor	146
Mediation of antibody dependent cellular cytotoxicity	152
Quantitation of serologic variables	
Immune complexes	156–159
Antibodies against infectious agents	160
Serum inhibitors of sheep erythrocyte binding to normal T-lymphocytes	137–139
IgG levels	149
Presence of autoantibodies	149
Anti T-lymphocyte antibodies	161
Lysozyme	7, 162–166, 180
Angiotensin-converting enzyme	7, 11, 131, 166–178, 180

SKIN TESTS AND BLOOD STUDIES

The mechanisms causing the anergic state in sarcoidosis are not well understood but probably involve circulating "factor(s)" that suppress the normal response of circulating inflammatory and immune effector cells to intradermal antigens (*see* Table 2). However, although anergy is a classic finding in pulmonary sarcoidosis (1, 3-5, 12, 19, 20, 133-143), there is no evidence that the anergic state reflects a concomitant high-intensity alveolitis or that normal skin test responses are characteristic of patients with low-intensity alveolitis (143-149). Likewise, although the numbers and function of blood mononuclear cells may have a broad correlation with disease activity, there is little evidence suggesting that such measurements accurately gauge the quantity and activity of the alveolitis of the sarcoid lung (23-29, 150-155).

The same reservations exist for most serologic tests proposed as monitors of disease activity. For example,

Table 3. Comparison of Proportions of T-Lymphocytes in Lavage Cell Differential with Biopsy Assessment of the Intensity of Alveolitis of Sarcoidosis Patients

Biopsy Assessment*	Percentages of T-Lymphocytes in the Lavage Cell Differential†	
	(≤28)	(>28)
Low-intensity alveolitis	6‡	0
High-intensity alveolitis	2	12‡

* Lung biopsies (approximately 1 cm by 1 cm, hemotoxylin and eosin stain), divided in a blinded fashion, were placed into a low- or high-intensity alveolitis group using criteria based on the number of mononuclear cells infiltrating the gas exchange exchange units (36).

† Patients were divided into two groups: those in whom lavage T-lymphocytes represented ≤28% of all inflammatory and immune effector cells present (low-intensity alveolitis) and those in whom T-lymphocutes represented >28% effector cells present (high-intensity alveolitis).

‡ The groupings of low-intensity alveolitis with ≤28% lavage T-lympnocytes and the high-intensity alveolitis with >28% lavage T-lymphocytes was significant at the $p < 0.01$ level.

there is no evidence that circulating immune complexes or various types of antibodies found in the serum of sarcoid patients are related to the inflammatory and immune processes within their lungs (156-161). However, two serologic variables, lysozyme and angiotensin-converting enzyme, should be considered because in theory, serum levels of these enzymes are linked to the class of phagocytic cells composing the alveolitis of sarcoidosis (11, 68, 162-180).

Lysozyme is an enzyme produced and secreted by many different cell types including cells of the mononuclear phagocytic series. In vitro, activated mononuclear phagocytes have an increased content of lysozyme and secrete more lysozyme into the culture medium (179). Thus, when the observation was made that patients with sarcoidosis frequently had increased levels of serum lysozyme, it was suggested that such measurements might reflect the activity of mononuclear phagocytes in these persons (68, 127, 163, 180). Several studies seem to support this concept. Blood monocytes of sarcoid patients secrete increased amounts of lysozyme compared to controls, monocyte lysozyme secretory rates correlate with the patient's lysozyme levels, and alveolar macrophages of these patients have more lysozyme activity than normal macrophages (68, 127).

Angiotensin-converting enzyme is generally regarded as a product of endothelial cells, where it acts to convert serum angiotensin I to angiotensin II and metabolizes bradykinin (181). However, when it was discovered that patients with sarcoidosis had increased serum levels of angiotensin-converting enzymes (168, 170), attention was directed toward the mechanism of this finding. Alveolar capillary endothelial cells seemed unlikely to be the source, because many chronic lung diseases are associated with injury to the alveolar capillary bed, yet increased angiotensin-converting enzyme levels are much commoner in sarcoidosis (11, 171). It was soon ascertained, however, that angiotensin-converting enzyme was present in lymph nodes, higher levels were present in nodes containing sarcoid granuloma (165), cells of the mononuclear phagocyte series contained and secreted angiotensin-converting enzyme (68, 128), and alveolar macrophages from sarcoid patients contained increased levels of this enzyme (68, 131). Thus, the concept evolved that cells of the mononuclear phagocyte series were the source of increased angiotensin-converting enzyme levels in sarcoidosis, and it was proposed that serum angiotensin-converting enzyme levels might reflect the inflammatory and immune processes in the lung parenchyma.

Unfortunately, in spite of the strong theoretical basis for the use of serum lysozyme and angiotensin-converting enzyme levels to gauge the activity of pulmonary sarcoidosis, there is conflicting evidence on the use of these variables in actually staging patients. Wheras some investigators have found that serum lysozyme and angiotensin-converting enzyme levels roughly correlate with disease activity (defined by symptoms or chest film) (11, 68, 131, 164, 166, 167, 169, 171-174), others have found either little or no correlation (168, 177) or have found that more patients with chronic disease than with acute disease have elevated levels (175). In addition, there have been no clinical studies showing a correlation of serum angiotensin-converting enzyme or lysozyme levels with the intensity of the alveolitis of sarcoidosis. In fact, there is direct evidence suggesting there is no correlation; quantitation of angiotensin-converting enzyme levels in lung parenchyma of sarcoid patients has shown them to be no different from those in normal persons (130, 131). Further confusing the picture is the observation that elevated serum angiotensin-converting enzyme levels also have been found in persons with disorders not involving the lungs, such as degenerative arthritis (171), cirrhosis (171), and granulomatous hepatitis (68, 169), suggesting that the quantity of this enzyme in the serum reflects a contribution from many organs. Because sarcoidosis is a systemic disease, the serum angiotensin-converting enzyme level probably reflects disease activity in many organs and has no specificity for disease activity within the alveolar structures.

In view of the above considerations, although it is clear that activated mononuclear phagocytes produce increased amounts of lysozyme and angiotensin converting enzyme, and that these cells are important components of the alveolitis of sarcoidosis, there is little evidence at present that these serum enzyme levels reflect the intensity of the alveolitis.

BRONCHOALVEOLAR LAVAGE

In contrast to the variables listed in Table 2, several lines of evidence support the concept that bronchoalveolar lavage is a useful clinical tool to sequentially measure the intensity of the inflammatory and immune processes within the alveolar structures of patients with pulmonary sarcoidosis.

1. As Dr. Hunninghake has discussed, bronchoalveolar lavage can be used to characterize the type and state of activation of the cells present within the alveolar structures (33). Although this method samples only cells on the epithelial surface of the lower respiratory tract, comparisons with analyses of effector cells in open lung biop-

sy specimens have shown that lavage analyses yield a representative average of the relative proportions of the various inflammatory and immune effector cells present throughout the alveolar structures (33, 65).

2. Even though lavage analyses are usually expressed in proportional terms (for example, proportion of all inflammatory and immune effector cells that are T-lymphocytes), comparison of lavage data with histologic data showed that for patients with pulmonary sarcoidosis, lavage analyses not only characterize the type of cells present but also estimate the overall intensity of the alveolitis (Table 3). To show this, we compared the proportions of T-lymphocytes recovered by lavage of a group of patients with sarcoidosis with a histologic estimate of the intensity of the alveolitis made by open lung biopsy. The biopsies, taken within 1 month of the lavage, were divided into two groups: those showing a high-intensity alveolitis (that is large numbers of mononuclear cells with the alveolar structures) and those showing a low-intensity alveolitis (that is, small numbers of mononuclear cells within the alveolar structures). Likewise, the lavage analyses were divided into two groups: those in which T-lymphocytes accounted for more than 28% of all cells recovered and those in which T-lymphocytes made up less than 28% of the effector cells present. Comparisons of these groupings showed a significant correlation between large numbers of mononuclear cells present in the biopsies and large proportions of T-lymphocytes recovered by lavage (65).

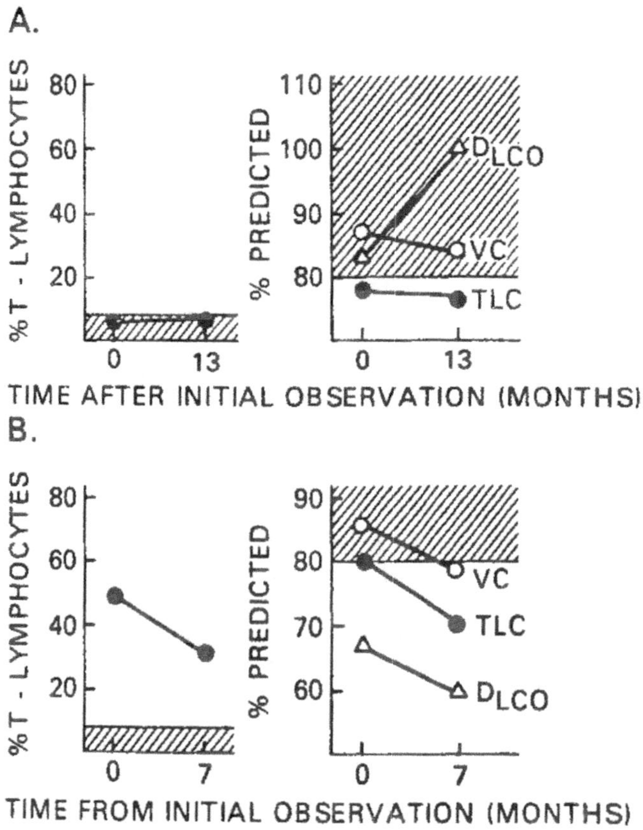

Figure 5. Prognostic use of bronchoalveolar lavage to evaluate the T-lymphocyte component of the alveolitis of pulmonary sarcoidosis. A. An untreated 22-year-old woman with pulmonary sarcoidosis seen over 13 months. During this period the alveolitis remained at a low level, and the pulmonary function variables remained stable or improved. B. An untreated 25-year-old woman with pulmonary sarcoidosis had a high-intensity alveolitis when first evaluated. After 7 months the alveolitis remained active, and all lung function variables had deteriorated. In both examples, the T-lymphocyte data are presented as the proportion of all lung effector cells that were T-lymphocytes, whereas the pulmonary function data are given in percent of predicted values. Shaded areas represent normal ranges. VC = vital capacity; TLC = total lung capacity; and D_{LCO} = single breath diffusing capacity (predicted based on alveolar volume and hemoglobin).

3. In our laboratories, bronchoalveolar lavage has been carried out in over 500 persons; it is associated with minimal discomfort, little morbidity, and no mortality (33). To ensure patient safety, however, it is important not to do lavage in patients with a forced expiratory volume in 1 s of less than 0.8 L. In addition, if inflammatory airway disease is present, lavage analyses must be interpreted cautiously, as it is difficult to estimate the relative contributions of bronchi and alveoli to the recovered cells.

4. Repeat lavage analyses over time show that in persons with pulmonary sarcoidosis in whom the proportion of T-lymphocytes remains low, there is little if any change in lung function over the same period (Figure 5A) (71). In contrast, for untreated patients in whom the proportion of lung T-lymphocytes remains high, lung function deteriorates (Figure 5B).

Such data support the concept that the alveolitis of sarcoidosis is a predecessor and cause of the anatomical derangements characteristic of sarcoidosis and that lavage is a useful monitor of the activity of the sarcoid alveolitis.

Roentgenograms and Physiologic Studies to Assess Activity

Dr. Jack D. Fulmer (Chief, Clinical Service, Pulmonary Branch, National Heart, Lung, and Blood Institute): The most commonly used monitors of pulmonary sarcoidosis are the chest roentgenogram and pulmonary function studies. Inherent in the use of these tests is the assumption that they help to stage the patient, that is, establish the extent and activity of the disease process, the prognosis, and the need for and efficacy of therapy. We will describe, therefore, the roentgenographic and physiologic findings in sarcoidosis and examine the available data concerning the sensitivity and specificity of these tests as monitors of disease activity. Also, because active pulmonary sarcoidosis is characterized by increased numbers of activated T-lymphocytes within the alveolar structures, we will evaluate the usefulness of the chest roentgenogram and common pulmonary function tests as detectors of the T-lymphocyte component of the alveolitis of this disease.

CHEST ROENTGENOGRAMS

The roentgenographic findings in pulmonary sarcoidosis have been well defined, and various classifications have been developed (12, 182-194). However, by international convention, the chest roentgenograms of patients with sarcoidosis are grouped according to the following scheme (12, 186): stage O, normal; stage I, bilateral hilar adenopathy; stage II, hilar adenopathy and diffuse parenchymal changes; and stage III, diffuse pulmonary infiltrates without hilar adenopathy. In this classification, the parenchymal changes most commonly described are fine or coarse nodules or a fluffy, cottonwood appearance; films with fibrotic changes, cysts, and bullae are usually assigned to stage III (12, 186). The proponents of this classification scheme view stages I through III as the roentgenographic manifestations of disease progression (186, 188). A worldwide review of 3676 patients with sarcoidosis showed that at the initial presentation to a physician, 8% had stage O roentgenograms, 51% had stage I, 29% had stage II, and 12% had stage III (186).

Although this international staging scheme is widely used in epidemiologic studies, most investigators believe that it often gives a false impression of the extent and activity of the disease process. Importantly, comparative morphologic-radiographic studies have shown that alveolitis and granulomas are present in the lung parenchyma of persons with stage I roentgenograms (5, 36, 195-198), even though the lung fields appear normal on the roentgenogram. In addition, although stage III roentgenograms are usually found only in those persons with progressive disease, it cannot be assumed that roentgenographic stages I and II always precede stage III (5).

To evaluate the usefulness of the classic roentgenographic staging in detecting the alveolitis in sarcoidosis, we categorized our study population into roentgenographic stages O to III and compared theses stages to estimates of the intensity of the alveolitis made from the lung biopsy. Consistent with the concept that the classic roentgenogram does not yield specific information concerning the activity of pulmonary sarcoidosis, no association was found between the roentgenographic stage and the quantitation of inflammatory and immune effector cells seen in the biopsy (33, 65). Further, comparison of the classic roentgenographic stages to the proportion of the T-lymphocytes recovered by bronchoalveolar lavage also showed no correlation.

In an attempt to escape the rigidity of the classic roentgenographic staging system, many investigators choose to simply describe the pattern seen; the most commonly described parenchymal patterns are reticulonodular, acinar, and fibrotic (189-192). Occasional patients also have large nodular lesions that simulate pulmonary metastasis, and cavitary lesions are sometimes found (184, 189, 193, 194). Although reticulonodular, acinar, and fibrotic patterns are widely recognized as manifestations of sarcoidosis, like the classic roentgenographic stages, their usefulness in staging the disease is unclear. It is generally accepted that the acinar and reticulonodular patterns precede the fibrotic pattern (189, 199, 200), but most evidence suggests that the chest film cannot be used to predict the morphologic findings (5, 36, 195, 201). Closely packed mononuclear cells within the alveolar air spaces have been suggested as the cause of the acinar pattern in sarcoidosis (191, 192), but there is also evidence that it is brought about by interstitial granulomas compressing the air spaces (190, 191). Attempts to correlate the alveolitis of sarcoidosis with these various roentgenographic presentations of sarcoidosis have failed. Evaluation of our study population also shows that there is little relation between the reticulonodular, acinar, and fibrotic patterns and the extent of alveolitis estimated by lung biopsy. Patients with acinar or nodular patterns generally had alveolitis and those with a coarse reticular pattern generally did not, but there was a great deal of overlap between groups. Likewise, no relationship could be found between the roentgenographic pattern and the proportion of bronchoalveolar lavage cells that were T-lymphocytes (33).

PHYSIOLOGIC TESTING

The usual physiologic findings in a patient with pulmonary sarcoidosis are characteristic of those of other patients with interstitial lung disease (3, 8, 189, 202-207). Lung volumes are reduced as are the diffusing capacity and lung compliance (202, 208-215). In addition, airway obstruction is a frequent physiologic finding in patients with sarcoidosis and seems to be unrelated to smoking history or the presence of bronchitis (8, 205, 206, 211, 215-223). Although many patients with sarcoidosis have a normal resting arterial oxygen tension, the resting alveolar-arterial oxygen gradient is often widened. In mild sarcoidosis, the arterial Po_2 may not change with exercise, but in persons with moderate and severe disease, increasing workloads cause the arterial oxygen tension to fall and the alveolar-arterial oxygen gradient to widen (8, 224-226).

Part of the problem in defining the functional consequences of sarcoidosis is that instead of using morphologic data as the standard for classifying patients, most investigators analyze the functional derangements from the perspective of the patient's roentgenographic stage (224). However, even though those with extensive roentgenographic changes usually have severe functional disturbances and those with minimal radiographic findings usually have few functional abnormalities (214), chest film and pulmonary function tests clearly have only a rough correlation to each other. A few studies have suggested that there is progressive impairment of pulmonary function with progressive roentgenographic changes (that is, stage I to III) (207), but for the majority of patients with sarcoidosis, most investigators have found little association between the chest film and physiologic tests (205, 211, 224, 227).

Functional testing is clearly more sensitive, however, to the disease process than the chest film. Many studies have shown examples of patients with stage I sarcoidosis who have abnormal diffusing capacity (189, 202, 207, 211, 224, 226). However, pulmonary function testing can be normal in the presence of parenchymal involvement (226, 227). Likewise, pulmonary function tests can be markedly abnormal but with the patient having little awareness of the functional derangement (228, 229).

As might be expected, some pulmonary function tests are more sensitive than others to this disease process. Measurements of lung volume are generally less sensitive than diffusing capacity, which in turn is less sensitive than gas exchange studies (particularly with exercise) (226, 227).

In our study population, comparison of the lung biopsy to the vital capacity, total lung capacity, diffusing capaci-

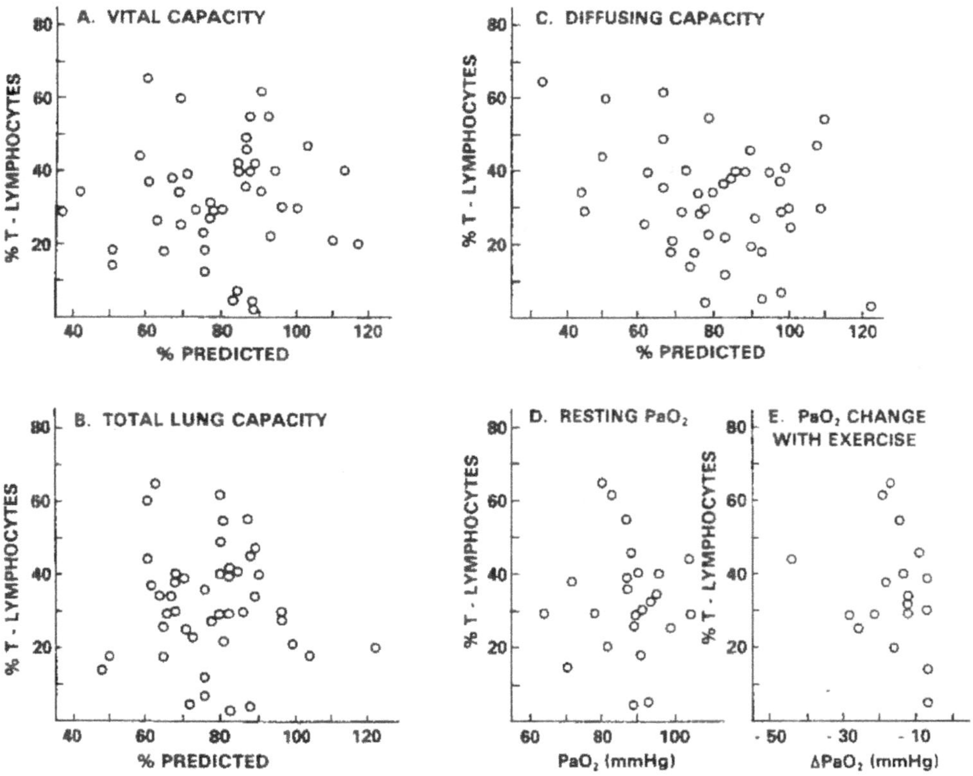

Figure 6. Evaluation of the ability of various pulmonary function variables to monitor the extent of the T-lymphocyte component of the alveolitis of sarcoidosis. The proportion of all lung effector cells that were T-lymphocytes (*% T-lymphocytes*) are compared to the percent predicted values for the following: **A.** Vital capacity. **B.** Total lung capacity. **C.** Single breath diffusing capacity (predicted based on alveolar volume and hemoglobin). **D.** Resting arterial oxygen tension. **E.** Change in arterial oxygen tension with exercise (PaO_2 [exercise]; PaO_2 [rest]).

ty, and resting exercising gas exchange data suggests that those studies are abnormal in the presence of alveolitis but cannot predict the extent of parenchymal inflammation. In addition, comparison of the proportion of T-lymphocytes in the lower respiratory tract to these variables showed that the magnitude of the functional abnormality has no relationship to the magnitude of the T-lymphocyte component of the alveolitis (Figure 6).

In summary, although radiographic and functional tests are useful to estimate the extent of disease within the alveolar structures, they cannot distinguish between alveolitis and anatomic derangement. Because the pathogenesis of the disease appears to be closely associated with the magnitude and characteristics of the alveolitis, we do not rely on roentgenographic and pulmonary function tests alone to make prognostic and therapeutic decisions in this disease (71).

Gallium Scanning to Assess Activity

Dr. Bruce R. Line (Senior Investigator, Department of Nuclear Medicine, Clinical Center and Laboratory of Applied Studies, Division of Computer Research and Technology): Gallium-67 (^{67}Ga) is a cyclotron-produced radionuclide with a half-life of 78 hours. This isotope was first used clinically to detect neoplastic disease (230-235). Soon thereafter, it was recognized that ^{67}Ga would also concentrate in sites of acute and chronic inflammation (231, 232, 235, 236). This property of ^{67}Ga is now widely used in the scintigraphic assessment of occult inflammation (237-245). It is thus natural to consider ^{67}Ga scanning as a noninvasive means of assessing the intensity of the alveolitis of sarcoidosis.

Gallium-67 scans are technically simple to do, cause no patient discomfort, and are associated with low radiation exposures (246, 247). The localization of ^{67}Ga in the region from the head to the pelvis is assessed from anterior and posterior rectilinear scans obtained 48 to 72 hours after intravenous administration of ^{67}Ga citrate (35 to 50 $\mu Ci/kg$). Normal lung tissue does not exceed the uptake of the nonspecific body background. Tissues that show significant physiologic uptake include the skeleton (spine, sternum, pelvis), the liver, and the spleen (Figure 7A) (248). To estimate the quality of ^{67}Ga taken up by lung alveolar tissues and minimize the effects of body structure and interpretive subjectivity, a semiquantitative "^{67}Ga-index" was devised (Figure 7) (249).

Abnormal gallium uptake in the lung is found in various pulmonary disorders with different pathogenesis and by itself is not diagnostic for any particular disease. Most categories of active interstitial lung disease have been associated with positive gallium scans (8). In some of these disorders, such as untreated idiopathic pulmonary fibrosis (249) and sarcoidosis (236, 242, 250, 251), positive gallium scans are the rule. In others, such as histiocytosis-X (LINE BR, FULMER JD, CRYSTAL RG. Unpublished observations), pulmonary uptake of ^{67}Ga is only occasionally observed. The reason for this wide range in sensitivity of the gallium scan is not clear but is probably associated with the type, intensity, and duration of the alveolitis of each disease.

GALLIUM SCANNING IN PULMONARY SARCOIDOSIS

A spectrum of ^{67}Ga uptake patterns can be found in the lungs of patients with sarcoidosis (Figure 7B to D). Diffuse mid- and lower lung zone parenchymal uptake are frequent, but focal or patchy localizations may be

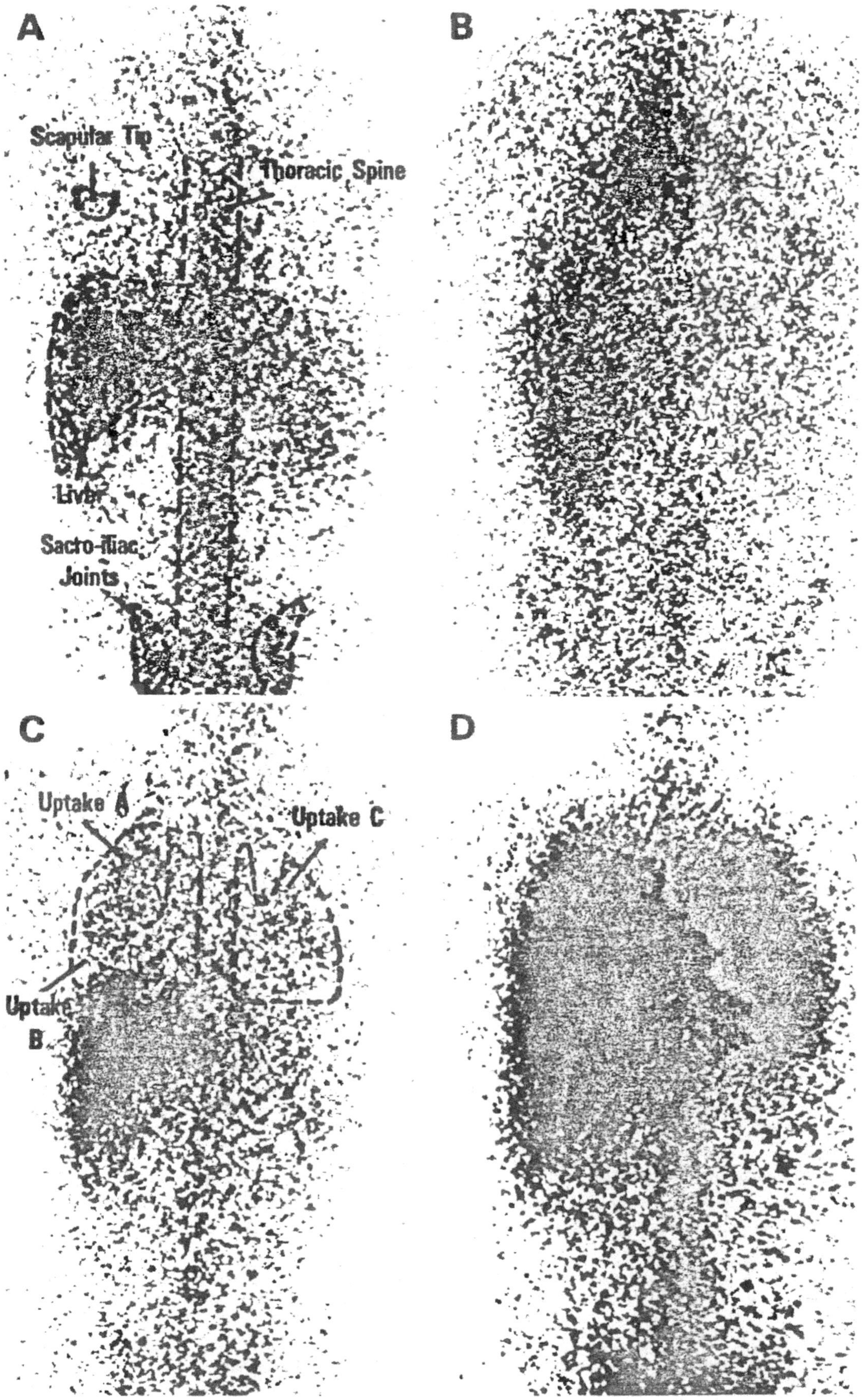

Figure 7. For Legend, see facing page.

present in any lung zone.

Although ^{67}Ga uptake is seen in other thoracic structures other than the lung parenchyma (such as hilar and paratracheal nodes), such uptake is not indicative of alveolitis and therefore not included in the computation of the parenchymal gallium uptake (249).

SIGNIFICANCE OF POSITIVE GALLIUM SCANS

The uptake of gallium in the lungs of patients with sarcoidosis is not associated with age, sex, smoking history, or duration of symptoms. In addition, there is no relation between the level of ^{67}Ga uptake and the functional status of the lung as assessed by lung volumes, by diffusing capacity, or by arterial blood gases at rest or with exercise.

To evaluate the usefulness of ^{67}Ga scans as an indicator of the alveolitis of sarcoidosis, we correlated ^{67}Ga-index estimates of pulmonary ^{67}Ga uptake with assessments of parenchymal inflammation by bronchoalveolar lavage. In the studies to date, there is a significant association of gallium uptake and the proportion of lung effector cells that are lymphocytes but an even stronger association of gallium uptake with the proportion of effector cells that were T-lymphocytes (unpublished observations). Because T-lymphocytes are important in the alveolitis of sarcoidosis, this evidence suggests that gallium uptake reflects the intensity of the T-lymphocyte component of the alveolitis. Consistent with the concept that T-lymphocytes may be responsible for ^{67}Ga uptake in sarcoidosis, Mertz and associates (252) showed in vitro that ^{67}Ga binds to the plasma membrane of lymphocytes. Further, the uptake was doubled when the lymphocytes were activated with phytohemagglutinin.

Further evidence for the usefulness of ^{67}Ga scans in assessing the alveolitis of sarcoidosis comes from the studies in Niden and associates (253) who showed good agreement between ^{67}Ga uptake and the presence of active inflammation in lung tissue obtained by biopsy. In addition, several studies have shown that parenchymal ^{67}Ga uptake is reduced when there is clinical remission of the disease (242, 250-252).

The spectrum of ^{67}Ga index in untreated patients with sarcoidosis (Figure 8) shows uptake scored from 10 to 340 units with indexes in more than two/thirds of patients above the normal limit of 50 units. Scans of untreated patients with sarcoid, compared to untreated patients with idiopathic pulmonary fibrosis, are generally more intense (Figure 8).

EXTRATHORACIC GALLIUM SCANNING

Although most interest in ^{67}Ga scanning in sarcoidosis has centered on the ^{67}Ga uptake by thoracic structures, gallium often localizes in extrathoracic tissues in this disease (Figures 9 and 10). As in the lung, ^{67}Ga uptake in extrathoracic structures is probably associated with increased proportions of T-lymphocytes. For example, the left iliac crest localization in the patient shown in Figure 10 was associated with larger than normal numbers of T-lymphocytes in the bone marrow of that region. In comparison, the iliac crest on the right did not take up gallium and has normal proportions of T-lymphocytes (28).

In summary, although not diagnostically specific, the ^{67}Ga scan can be used to repetitively characterize the severity and anatomic location of regions of alveolitis and can provide a longitudinal assessment of the degree of inflammation in the whole parenchyma. Gallium-67 scanning is available, noninvasive, and involves low radi-

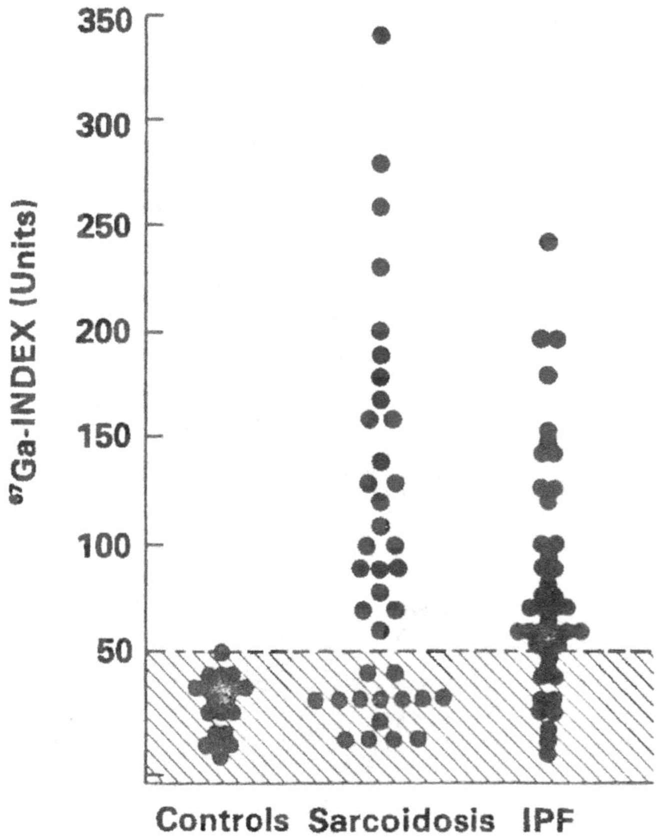

Figure 8. Distribution of ^{67}Ga index in control patients and in untreated patients with sarcoidosis and idiopathic pulmonary fibrosis (*IPF*). All control scans show ^{67}Ga index values below 50 ^{67}Ga index units. Sixty-three percent of the untreated patients with sarcoidosis show ^{67}Ga index values greater than 50 index units. In contrast, 74% of the untreated patients with idiopathic pulmonary fibrosis have ^{67}Ga index values greater than 50 index units (249). As a group, untreated patients with sarcoidosis show greater gallium lung uptake than do untreated patients with idiopathic pulmonary fibrosis. Shaded area represents normal range.

Figure 7. Examples of ^{67}Ga index computation in a normal person and in three patients with pulmonary sarcoidosis; the method used to quantitate the ^{67}Ga index is as outlined in reference 249. **A.** Normal scan in a 36-year-old man showing physiologic ^{67}Ga uptake in skeletal tissues (scapular tips, spine, pelvis, sacroiliac joints), liver, and spleen. Localization in the pulmonary parenchyma is similar to background (estimated from uptake in abdominal region below kidneys). Gallium-67 index = 10 index units. **B.** Scan of 45-year-old woman with pulmonary sarcoidosis showing right paratracheal and bilateral hilar nodal uptake and mild lower lung zone ^{67}Ga uptake (intensity = 1, area = 30%, equivalent to a ^{67}Ga index of 30 units. **C.** Scan of a 42-year-old man with pulmonary sarcoidosis. Three regions show uptake greater than the background area. Region A (intensity = 2, area = 20%, index = 40 units), region B (intensity = 1 area = 20%, index = 20 units), and region C (intensity = 1, area = 30%, index = 30 units) are summed to give a total ^{67}Ga index of 90 units. **D.** Diffuse high intensity ^{67}Ga uptake in a 36-year-old man with pulmonary sarcoidosis. The ^{67}Ga index is equivalent to 340 units.

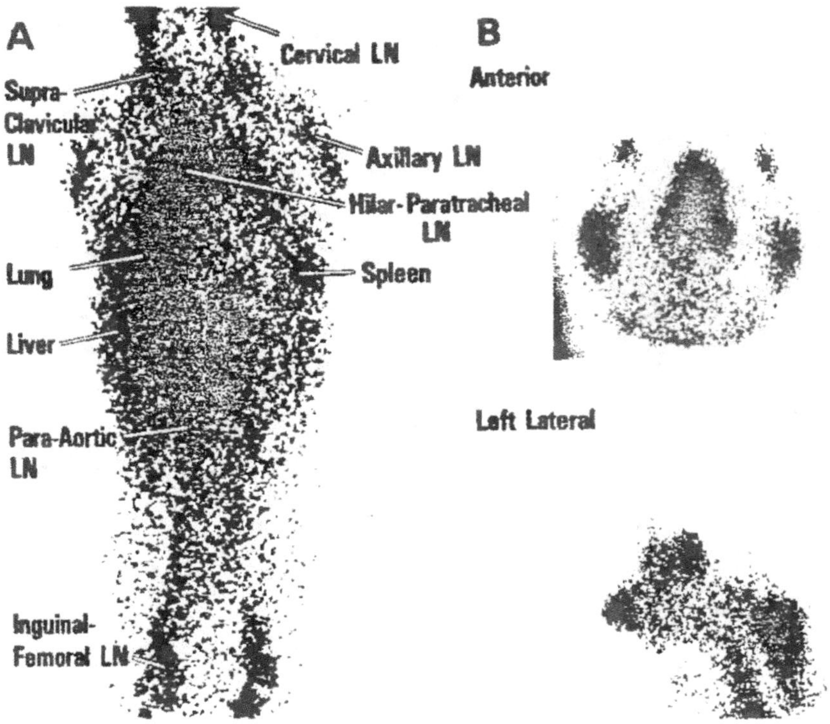

Figure 9. Extrathoracic ^{67}Ga localization in sarcoidosis. **A.** Sarcoidosis in 32-year-old woman. Gallium localization is noted in cervical, supraclavicular, axillary, mediastinal, para-aortic, inguinal, and femoral lymph nodes (*LN*) and in pulmonary parenchyma at base of right lung. **B.** Nasopharyngeal and parotid gland uptake of ^{67}Ga in 24-year-old man with sarcoidosis. There was clinical evidence of sarcoidosis of the nasopharynx but not of the parotids.

ation exposures. It should prove useful in staging patients with sarcoidosis and in following their response to therapy.

Treatment of Pulmonary Sarcoidosis

Dr. Ronald G. Crystal: Although the cause of pulmonary sarcoidosis is unknown, the disease clearly is characterized and perpetuated by activated T-lymphocytes within the alveolar structures. This is probably only part of the picture. For example, an important effector role will probably be found for mononuclear phagocytes in the lung other than simply as building blocks for granuloma formation. However, the knowledge that activated lung T-lymphocytes play a central role in the pathogenesis of this disease permits a rational assessment of therapeutic strategies.

CORTICOSTEROID THERAPY

Corticosteroids are the principal therapy against sarcoidosis. During the past 25 years, the following concepts have emerged (1, 3, 5, 7, 13, 15, 16, 35, 215, 254-261): [1] Corticosteroids generally improve symptoms, may or may not improve roentgenographic abnormalities, and variably improve lung function. [2] To be effective, corticosteroids must be given early and for at least 3 to 6 months. When they are withdrawn, relapses are frequent. Although long-term corticosteroid therapy seems to benefit most patients, the conditions of a small proportion will still deteriorate. [3] If low doses are used for maintenance therapy (for example, prednisone $\leq$ 0.25 mg/kg of body weight a day), complications are infrequent and mild.

Most of these observations are consistent with the concept that corticosteroids suppress the alveolitis of sarcoidosis but have little direct influence on the anatomic derangements of the alveolar structures that occurred before the institution of therapy. In humans, corticosteroids impair T-lymphocyte proliferation (262-264) and T-cell effector functions (265-266). They may affect the distribution of immune effector cells, including the proportioning of T-lymphocytes between blood and various organs (267, 268). These agents also have a profound effect on the capacity of mononuclear phagocytes to respond to mediators produced by T-lymphocytes (269). Thus it is reasonable to hypothesize that when corticosteroids are given in appropriate doses to patients with pulmonary sarcoidosis, they should prevent T-lymphocyte-mediated recruitment of blood monocytes to the lung and thus inhibit granuloma formation. Also, because granulomas are dynamic structures (85, 88), the reduction in recruitment of blood monocytes probably will cause a reduction in the number and size of existing granulomas.

Because both the alveolitis and granulomas impair lung function, therapy with corticosteroids should improve lung function by reducing the intensity of the alveolitis and reducing the lung burden of granuloma. In addition, by suppressing the alveolitis, corticosteroids prevent future derangements of the alveolar structures. However, there is no evidence that corticosteroids can improve interstitial fibrosis or alterations in lung parenchymal cells once present, that is, a deranged alveolus cannot be rebuilt and is lost forever as a gas-exchanging unit (270, 271).

Generally, studies evaluating the efficacy of corticosteriods in pulmonary sarcoidosis have relied on one or more of the following criteria as evidence for a beneficial therapeutic effect: a reduction in symptoms related to the lungs, particularly dyspnea; improvement in the chest roentgenogram; and improvement in functional tests such as lung volumes, diffusing capacity, and arterial

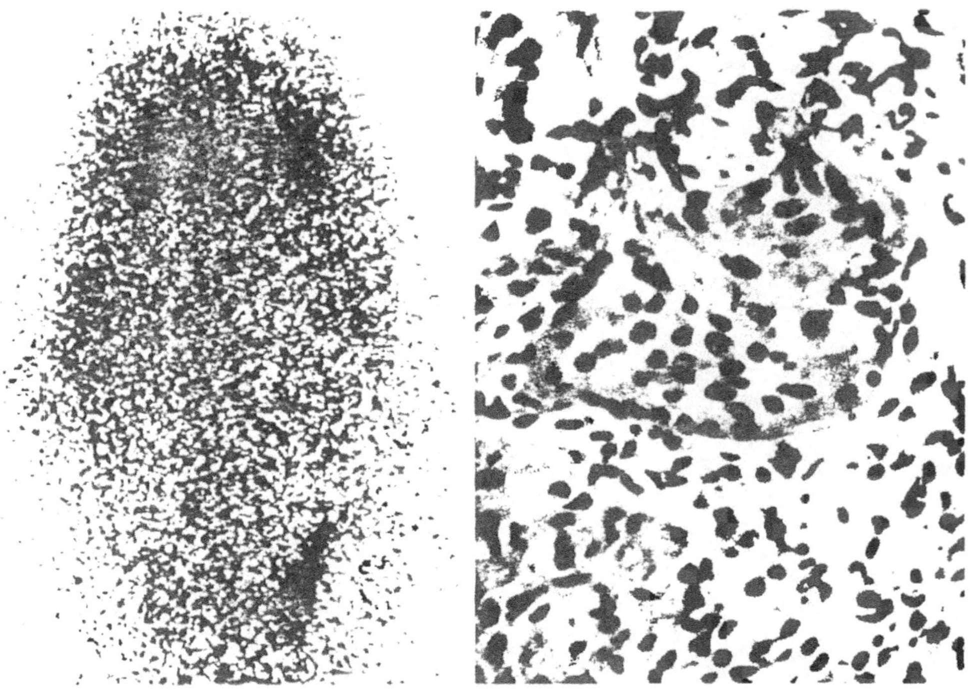

Figure 10 **Left.** Extrathoracic uptake in left posterior iliac crest of a 63-year-old man. There is also diffuse parenchymal ^{67}Ga uptake with right apical prominence and mediastinal-bilateral hilar node involvement. **Right.** Biopsy of left posterior iliac crest of the patient in left-hand panel showing noncaseating granulomas consistent with sarcoidosis.

blood gases at rest and during exercise. However, in view of our previous discussions, the difficulty assessing the efficacy of corticosteroids using these variables is understandable. Corticosteroids act on the alveolitis, not the derangements of the alveolar structures, yet there have been no studies comparing pulmonary symptoms to the intensity of the alveolitis or the anatomic derangements of the alveolar structures; the chest roentgenogram cannot clearly distinguish between alveolitis and anatomic derangement and is relatively insensitive to the presence of alveolitis; and because functional tests probably detect alveolitis as well as granulomas, fibrosis, and other derangements of the alveolar structures, they cannot be used to follow change in the alveolitis. Thus, even if corticosteroids were to effectively reduce the proportion of T-lymphocytes within the lung of a person with sarcoidosis, this beneficial effect may not be detected by the conventional monitors of the disease process. Because both alveolitis and anatomic derangements seem to influence radiographic and functional tests, an improvement in the alveolitis may be masked by a stabilized, but abnormal, anatomic arrangement of the alveolar structures.

THERAPY OF SARCOIDOSIS: OTHER AGENTS

Besides corticosteroids, chloroquine (272), D-penacillamine (273), spirononolactone (274), allopurinol (275), levamisole (276), heparin (277), and phenylbutazone (278) have also been used in the therapy of sarcoidosis. Except for chloroquine, none have been evaluated by controlled trials, and the results with chloroquine are equivocal (272). In view of the current concepts of the disease, there is little theoretical basis for the use of any of these agents. Cytotoxic agents such as chlorambucil (279), azathioprine (280), and methotrexate (279) have also been used, but only in a few patients. No controls were used, the patients were mostly those with advanced disease, and the effect of these drugs on the alveolitis was not evaluated. Thus, although such drugs might suppress lung T-lymphocytes, at this time they cannot be considered as tested therapies for this disease.

FUTURE APPROACHES

The observations that T-lymphocytes play an important role in the pathogenesis of pulmonary sarcoidosis and that the alveolitis of this disease precedes anatomic derangements in the alveolar structures suggest that monitors of lung T-lymphocyte number may provide a convenient and logical guide to therapy decisions and the assessment of new treatment protocols.

ACKNOWLEDGMENTS: The authors thank Drs. Gordon Head and Andrew Dwyer of the Radiology Department, Clinical Center, National Institutes of Health, for assistance in classifying the chest radiographs; Charlotte Kenton of the National Library of Medicine for invaluable help in searching the extensive sarcoidosis literature; and Mrs. Lou West and Mrs. Ellen Wright for excellent editorial assistance.

▶ Requests for reprints should be addressed to Ronald G. Crystal, M.D.; Building 10, Room 6D06, National Institutes of Health; Bethesda, MD 20205.

References

1. Scadding JG. *Sarcoidosis.* London: Eyre and Spottiswoode Ltd.; 1967.
2. Spencer H. *Pathology of the Lung.* New York: Pergammon Press; 1977.
3. Crofton J, Douglas A. *Respiratory Disease.* Oxford: Blackwell Scientific Publications; 1975.
4. Fraser RG, Paré JAP. *Diagnosis of Diseases of the Chest.* Philadelphia: W. B. Saunders Co.; 1979.
5. Mitchell DN, Scadding JG. Sarcoidosis. *Am Rev Respir Dis.* 1974;110:774-802.
6. Mitchell DN, Scadding JG, Heard BE, et al. Sarcoidosis: histopathological definition and clinical diagnosis. *J Clin Pathol.* 1977;30:395-408.
7. Israel H. Sarcoidosis. In: Simmons DH, ed. *Current Pulmonology.* Vol. 1. Boston: Houghton Mifflin; 1979:163-82.
8. Fulmer JD, Crystal RG. Interstitial lung disease. In: Simmons DH, ed. *Current Pulmonology.* Vol. 1. Boston: Houghton Mifflin; 1979:1-65.
9. Kent DC, Houk VN, Elliott RC, Sokolowski JW Jr, Baker JH,

Sorensen K. The definitive evaluation of sarcoidosis. *Am Rev Respir Dis.* 1970;**101**:721-7.

10. Koerner SK, Sakowitz AJ, Appelman RI, Becker NH, Schoenbaum SW. Transbronchial lung biopsy for the diagnosis of sarcoidosis. *N Engl J Med.* 1975;**293**:268-70.
11. Lieberman J, Nosal A, Schlessner L, Sastre-Foken A. Serum angiotensin-converting enzyme for diagnosis and therapeutic evaluation of sarcoidosis. *Am Rev Respir Dis.* 1979;**120**:329-35.
12. Siltzbach LE, James DG, Neville E, et al. Course and prognosis of sarcoidosis around the world. *Am J Med.* 1974;**57**:847-52.
13. James DG, Neville E, Siltzbach LE, et al. A worldwide survey of sarcoid. In: Siltzbach LE, ed. Seventh International Conference on Sarcoidosis. *Ann NY Acad Sci.* 1976;**278**:321-34.
14. Mayock RL, Bertrand P, Morrison CE, Scott JH. Manifestations of sarcoidosis: analysis of 145 patients with a review of 9 series selected from the literature. *Am J Med.* 1963;**35**:67-89.
15. Israel HL. Prognosis of sarcoidosis. *Ann Intern Med.* 1970;**73**:1038-9.
16. Sones M, Israel HL. Course and prognosis of sarcoidosis. *Am J Med.* 1960;**28**:84-93.
17. Bacharach T. Sarcoidosis: a clinical review of 111 cases. *Am Rev Respir Dis.* 1961;**84**:12-6.
18. Longcope WT, Freiman DG. A study of sarcoidosis. *Medicine (Baltimore).* 1952;**31**:1-132.
19. Geraint-James D. Immunology of sarcoidosis. *Lancet.* 1966;**2**:633-4.
20. Sones M, Israel HC. Altered immunologic reactions in sarcoidosis.
21. Hirschorn K, Schreibman RR, Bach FH et al. *In vitro* studies of lymphocytes from patients with sarcoidosis and lymphoproliferative diseases. *Lancet.* 1964;**2**:842-3.
22. Sharma OP, James DG, Fox RA. A correlation of *in vitro* delayed type hypersensitivity and *in vitro* lymphocyte transformation in sarcoidosis. *Chest.* 1971;**60**:35-7.
23. Kataria YP, Sagone AL, LoBuglio AF, et al. *In vitro* observations on sarcoid lymphocytes and their correlation with cutaneous anergy and clinical severity of disease. *Am Rev Respir Dis.* 1973;**108**:767-76.
24. Hedfors E, Holm G, Petterson E. Lymphocyte subpopulations in sarcoidosis. *Clin Exp Immunol.* 1974;**17**:219-26.
25. Daniele RP, Rowlands DT Jr. Lymphocyte subpopulations in sarcoidosis: correlation with disease activity and duration. *Ann Intern Med.* 1976;**85**:593-600.
26. Ramachandar K, Douglas SD, Siltzbach LE, et al. Peripheral blood lymphocyte subpopulations in sarcoidosis. *Cell Immunol.* 1975;**16**:422-6.
27. Sorensen SF, Hardt F, Veien NF. Estimation of lymphocyte subpopulations in peripheral blood of patients with sarcoidosis. *Scand J Immunol.* 1976;**5**:117-22.
28. Hunninghake GW, Fulmer JD, Young RC Jr, Gadek JE, Crystal RG. Localization of the immune response in sarcoidosis. *Am Rev Respir Dis.* 1979;**120**:49-57.
29. Hunninghake G, Kelman J, Weinberger S, Young R, Fulmer J, Crystal RG. Lung lymphocyte subpopulations in sarcoidosis. *Clin Res.* 1978;**26**:448A. Abstract.
30. Hunninghake GW, Kelman JA, Gadek JE, Elson NA, Fulmer JD, Crystal RG. Comparison of inflammatory and immune effector cell populations in lavage fluid and lung biopsies of patients with pulmonary fibrosis. *Am Rev Respir Dis.* 1978;**177** (suppl): 68. Abstract.
31. Hunninghake G, Gadek J, Weinberger S, et al. Comparison of the alveolitis of sarcoidosis and idiopathic pulmonary fibrosis. *Chest.* 1979;**75S**:266S-67S.
32. Hunninghake GW, Fulmer JD, Young RC, Crystal RG. Comparison of lung and blood lymphocyte subpopulations in pulmonary sarcoidosis. In: Williams, WJ, Davies, BH, eds. *Proceedings of the 8th International Conference on Sarcoidosis and Other Granulomatous Disease.* London: Alpha Omega Publishing, Ltd.; 1980:426-35.
33. Hunninghake GW, Gadek JE, Kawanami O, Ferrans VJ, Crystal RG. Inflammatory and immune processes in the human lung in health and disease: evaluation by bronchoalveolar lavage. *Am J Pathol.* 1979;**97**:149-206.
34. Hunninghake GW, Gadek JE, Young RC Jr, Kawanami O, Ferrans VJ, Crystal RG. Mechanisms of granuloma formation in pulmonary sarcoidosis by T-lymphocytes within the lung. *N Engl J Med.* 1980;**302**:594-8.
35. Siltzbach LE. Sarcoidosis. In: Fishman AP, ed. *Pulmonary Diseases and Disorders.* New York: McGraw-Hill; 1980:899-908.
36. Carrington CB, Gaensler EA, Milsus JP, et al. Structure and function in sarcoidosis. *Ann NY Acad Sci.* 1976;**278**:265-82.
37. Soler P, Basset F. Morphology and distribution of the cells of a sarcoid granuloma: ultrastructural study of serial sections. *Ann NY Acad Sci.* 1976;**278**:147-60.
38. Soler P, Bernaudin JF, Basset F, Basset G. Epithelioid cell and sarcoid-like granuloma: a review of human and experimental material. *Mt Sinai J Med.* 1977;**44**:767-71.
39. Van Furth R. Origin and kinetics of monocytes and macrophages. *Semin Hematol.* 1970;**7**:125-41.
40. James EM, Williams WJ. Fine structure and histochemistry of epithelioid cells in sarcoidosis. *Thorax.* 1974;**29**:115-20.
41. Wanstrup J, Christensen HE. Sarcoidosis: I. Ultrastructural investigations on epithelioid cell granulomas. *Acta Pathol Microbiol Scand.* 1966;**66**:169-85.
42. Jones-Williams W, Erazmus DA, Valerie-James EM, Davies T. The fine structure of sarcoid and tuberculous granulomas. *Postgrad Med J.* 1970;**46**:496-500.
43. Fuse Y, Hiragi Y. The fine structures of sarcoidal and Kveim granulomas. In: Iwai K, Hasodo Y, eds. *Proceedings of the VI International Conference on Sarcoidosis.* Baltimore: University Park Press; 1974;269-75.
44. Fukushiro R, Hirone T, Eryn Y. Ultrastructural and cytochemical observations on sarcoid granulomas. In: Levinsky L, Macholda F, eds. *Fifth International Conference on Sarcoidosis.* Prague: Universita Karlova; 1971:276-9.
45. Carr I, Norris P. The fine structure of human machrophage granules in sarcoidosis. *J Pathol.* 1977;**122**:29-32.
46. Biberfield P. Morphogenesis in blood lymphocytes stimulated with phytohaemagglutinin (PITA): a light and electron microscopic study. *Acta Pathol Microbiol Scand [A].* **223** (suppl):1-70.
47. Teilum G. Allergic hyperglobulinosis and hyalinosis (paraamyloidosis) in the reticulo-endothelial system in Boecks sarcoid and other conditions: a morphologic immunity reaction. *Am J Pathol.* 1948;**24**:389-407.
48. Kalifat SR, Bouteille M, Belarue J. Changes in connective tissue in sarcoid granuloma: hyalin, paraamyloid and fibrinoid: electron microscopic study of 11 cases. *Virchows Arch Abt B Zellpath.* 1969;**3**:348-58.
49. Weinberger SE, Crystal RG. Reactions of the interstitial space to injury. In: Fishman AP, ed. *Pulmonary Diseases and Disorders.* New York: McGraw-Hill; 1980;640-7.
50. Divertie MB, Cassan SM, Brown AL. Ultrastructural morphometry of blood-air barrier in pulmonary sarcoidosis. *Chest.* 1976;**69**:154-7.
51. Pinner M. Noncaseating tuberculosis. *Am Rev Tuberc.* 1938;**37**:690-728.
52. Rosen Y, Athanassiades TJ, Moon S, et al. Nongranulomatous interstitial pneumonitis in sarcoidosis: relationship to the development of epithelioid granulomas. *Chest.* 1978;**74**:122-5.
53. Takahashi M. Histopathology of sarcoidosis and its immunological basis. *Acta Pathol Jpn.* 1970;**20**:171-82.
54. Teilum G. Morphogenesis and development of sarcoid lesions: similarities to the group of collagenosis. *Acta Med Scand.* 1964;**425** (suppl):14-8.
55. Judd PA, Finnegan P, Curran RC. Pulmonary sarcoidosis: a clinicopathologic study. *J Pathol.* 1975;**115**:191-8.
56. Cain H, Kraus B. Asteroid bodies: derivatives of the cytosphere. *Virchows Arch [Cell Pathol].* 1977;**26**:119-32.
57. Obel AL, Löfgren S. Pathogenesis of hyaline formation in sarcoidosis lymph nodes. *Acta Med Scand.* 1964;**425**(suppl):27-30.
58. DiBenedetto RJ, Ribaudo C. Bronchopulmonary sarcoidosis. *Am Rev Respir Dis.* 1966;**94**:952-5.
59. Scadding JG. The late stages of pulmonary sarcoidosis. *Postgrad Med J.* 1970;**46**:530-6.
60. Boros OL. Granulomatous inflammations. *Prog Allergy.* 1978;**24**:183-267.
61. Reynolds HY, Newball HH. Analysis of proteins and respiratory cells obtained from human lungs by bronchial lavage. *J Lab Clin Med.* 1974;**84**:559-73.
62. Reynolds HY, Fulmer JD Kazmierowski JA, Roberts WC, Frank MM, Crystal RG. Analysis of bronchoalveolar lavage fluid from patients with idiopathic pulmonary fibrosis and chronic hypersensitivity pneumonitis. *J Clin Invest.* 1977;**59**:165-75.
63. Weinberger SE, Kelman JA, Elson NA, et al. Bronchoalveolar lavage in interstitial lung disease. *Ann Intern Med.* 1978;**89**:459-66.
64. Hunninghake GW, Gadek JE, Szapiel SV, et al. The human alveolar macrophage. In: Harris CC, Trump BF, Stoner GD, eds. *Cultured Human Cells and Tissues in Bio-Medical Research.* New York: Academic Press; 1980. *(Methods and Perspectives in Cell Biology,* Vol. 1).
65. Hunninghake GW, Kawanami O, Ferrans VI, et al. Characterization of the inflammatory and immune effector cells in lung parenchyma of patients with interstitial lung disease. *Am Rev Respir Dis.* In press.
66. Yeager J, Williams MC, Beekman JF, Bayly TC, Beaman BL, Hawley RJ. Sarcoidosis: analysis of cells obtained by bronchial lavage. *Am Rev Respir Dis.* 1977;**116**:951-5.
67. Reynolds HY. The importance of lymphocytes in pulmonary health and disease. *Lung.* 1978;**155**:225-42.
68. Gee JB, Godel PT, Zorn SK, et al. Sarcoidosis and mononuclear

Sorensen K. The definitive evaluation of sarcoidosis. *Am Rev Respir Dis.* 1970;**101**:721-7.
10. Koerner SK, Sakowitz AJ, Appelman RI, Becker NH, Schoenbaum SW. Transbronchial lung biopsy for the diagnosis of sarcoidosis. *N Engl J Med.* 1975;**293**:268-70.
11. Lieberman J, Nosal A, Schlessner L, Sastre-Foken A. Serum angiotensin-converting enzyme for diagnosis and therapeutic evaluation of sarcoidosis. *Am Rev Respir Dis.* 1979;**120**:329-35.
12. Siltzbach LE, James DG, Neville E, et al. Course and prognosis of sarcoidosis around the world. *Am J Med.* 1974;**57**:847-52.
13. James DG, Neville E, Siltzbach LE, et al. A worldwide survey of sarcoid. In: Siltzbach LE, ed. Seventh International Conference on Sarcoidosis. *Ann NY Acad Sci.* 1976;**278**:321-34.
14. Mayock RL, Bertrand P, Morrison CE, Scott JH. Manifestations of sarcoidosis: analysis of 145 patients with a review of 9 series selected from the literature. *Am J Med.* 1963;**35**:67-89.
15. Israel HL. Prognosis of sarcoidosis. *Ann Intern Med.* 1970;**73**:1038-9.
16. Sones M, Israel HL. Course and prognosis of sarcoidosis. *Am J Med.* 1960;**28**:84-93.
17. Bacharach T. Sarcoidosis: a clinical review of 111 cases. *Am Rev Respir Dis.* 1961;**84**:12-6.
18. Longcope WT, Freiman DG. A study of sarcoidosis. *Medicine (Baltimore).* 1952;**31**:1-132.
19. Geraint-James D. Immunology of sarcoidosis. *Lancet.* 1966;**2**:633-4.
20. Sones M, Israel HC. Altered immunologic reactions in sarcoidosis.
21. Hirschorn K, Schreibman RR, Bach FH et al. *In vitro* studies of lymphocytes from patients with sarcoidosis and lymphoproliferative diseases. *Lancet.* 1964;**2**:842-3.
22. Sharma OP, James DG, Fox RA. A correlation of *in vitro* delayed type hypersensitivity and *in vitro* lymphocyte transformation in sarcoidosis. *Chest.* 1971;**60**:35-7.
23. Kataria YP, Sagone AL, LoBuglio AF, et al. *In vitro* observations on sarcoid lymphocytes and their correlation with cutaneous anergy and clinical severity of disease. *Am Rev Respir Dis.* 1973;**108**:767-76.
24. Hedfors E, Holm G, Petterson E. Lymphocyte subpopulations in sarcoidosis. *Clin Exp Immunol.* 1974;**17**:219-26.
25. Daniele RP, Rowlands DT Jr. Lymphocyte subpopulations in sarcoidosis: correlation with disease activity and duration. *Ann Intern Med.* 1976;**85**:593-600.
26. Ramachandar K, Douglas SD, Siltzbach LE, et al. Peripheral blood lymphocyte subpopulations in sarcoidosis. *Cell Immunol.* 1975;**16**:422-6.
27. Sorensen SF, Hardt F, Veien NF. Estimation of lymphocyte subpopulations in peripheral blood of patients with sarcoidosis. *Scand J Immunol.* 1976;**5**:117-22.
28. Hunninghake GW, Fulmer JD, Young RC Jr, Gadek JE, Crystal RG. Localization of the immune response in sarcoidosis. *Am Rev Respir Dis.* 1979;**120**:49-57.
29. Hunninghake G, Kelman J, Weinberger S, Young R, Fulmer J, Crystal RG. Lung lymphocyte subpopulations in sarcoidosis. *Clin Res.* 1978;**26**:448A. Abstract.
30. Hunninghake GW, Kelman JA, Gadek JE, Elson NA, Fulmer JD, Crystal RG. Comparison of inflammatory and immune effector cell populations in lavage fluid and lung biopsies of patients with pulmonary fibrosis. *Am Rev Respir Dis.* 1978;**177** (suppl): 68. Abstract.
31. Hunninghake G, Gadek J, Weinberger S, et al. Comparison of the alveolitis of sarcoidosis and idiopathic pulmonary fibrosis. *Chest.* 1979;**75S**:266S-67S.
32. Hunninghake GW, Fulmer JD, Young RC, Crystal RG. Comparison of lung and blood lymphocyte subpopulations in pulmonary sarcoidosis. In: Williams, WJ, Davies, BH, eds. *Proceedings of the 8th International Conference on Sarcoidosis and Other Granulomatous Disease.* London: Alpha Omega Publishing, Ltd.; 1980:426-35.
33. Hunninghake GW, Gadek JE, Kawanami O, Ferrans VJ, Crystal RG. Inflammatory and immune processes in the human lung in health and disease: evaluation by bronchoalveolar lavage. *Am J Pathol.* 1979;**97**:149-206.
34. Hunninghake GW, Gadek JE, Young RC Jr, Kawanami O, Ferrans VJ, Crystal RG. Mechanisms of granuloma formation in pulmonary sarcoidosis by T-lymphocytes within the lung. *N Engl J Med.* 1980;**302**:594-8.
35. Siltzbach LE. Sarcoidosis. In: Fishman AP, ed. *Pulmonary Diseases and Disorders.* New York: McGraw-Hill; 1980:899-908.
36. Carrington CB, Gaensler EA, Milsus JP, et al. Structure and function in sarcoidosis. *Ann NY Acad Sci.* 1976;**278**:265-82.
37. Soler P, Basset F. Morphology and distribution of the cells of a sarcoid granuloma: ultrastructural study of serial sections. *Ann NY Acad Sci.* 1976;**278**:147-60.
38. Soler P, Bernaudin JF, Basset F, Basset G. Epithelioid cell and sarcoid-like granuloma: a review of human and experimental material. *Mt Sinai J Med.* 1977;**44**:767-71.
39. Van Furth R. Origin and kinetics of monocytes and macrophages. *Semin Hematol.* 1970;**7**:125-41.
40. James EM, Williams WJ. Fine structure and histochemistry of epithelioid cells in sarcoidosis. *Thorax.* 1974;**29**:115-20.
41. Wanstrup J, Christensen HE. Sarcoidosis: I. Ultrastructural investigations on epithelioid cell granulomas. *Acta Pathol Microbiol Scand.* 1966;**66**:169-85.
42. Jones-Williams W, Erazmus DA, Valerie-James EM, Davies T. The fine structure of sarcoid and tuberculous granulomas. *Postgrad Med J.* 1970;**46**:496-500.
43. Fuse Y, Hiragi Y. The fine structures of sarcoidal and Kveim granulomas. In: Iwai K, Hasodo Y, eds. *Proceedings of the VI International Conference on Sarcoidosis.* Baltimore: University Park Press; 1974;269-75.
44. Fukushiro R, Hirone T, Eryn Y. Ultrastructural and cytochemical observations on sarcoid granulomas. In: Levinsky L, Macholda F, eds. *Fifth International Conference on Sarcoidosis.* Prague: Universita Karlova; 1971:276-9.
45. Carr I, Norris P. The fine structure of human machrophage granules in sarcoidosis. *J Pathol.* 1977;**122**:29-32.
46. Biberfield P. Morphogenesis in blood lymphocytes stimulated with phytohaemagglutinin (PITA): a light and electron microscopic study. *Acta Pathol Microbiol Scand [A].* **223** (suppl):1-70.
47. Teilum G. Allergic hyperglobulinosis and hyalinosis (paraamyloidosis) in the reticulo-endothelial system in Boecks sarcoid and other conditions: a morphologic immunity reaction. *Am J Pathol.* 1948;**24**:389-407.
48. Kalifat SR, Bouteille M, Belarue J. Changes in connective tissue in sarcoid granuloma: hyalin, paraamyloid and fibrinoid: electron microscopic study of 11 cases. *Virchows Arch Abt B Zellpath.* 1969;**3**:348-58.
49. Weinberger SE, Crystal RG. Reactions of the interstitial space to injury. In: Fishman AP, ed. *Pulmonary Diseases and Disorders.* New York: McGraw-Hill; 1980;640-7.
50. Divertie MB, Cassan SM, Brown AL. Ultrastructural morphometry of blood-air barrier in pulmonary sarcoidosis. *Chest.* 1976;**69**:154-7.
51. Pinner M. Noncaseating tuberculosis. *Am Rev Tuberc.* 1938;**37**:690-728.
52. Rosen Y, Athanassiades TJ, Moon S, et al. Nongranulomatous interstitial pneumonitis in sarcoidosis: relationship to the development of epithelioid granulomas. *Chest.* 1978;**74**:122-5.
53. Takahashi M. Histopathology of sarcoidosis and its immunological basis. *Acta Pathol Jpn.* 1970;**20**:171-82.
54. Teilum G. Morphogenesis and development of sarcoid lesions: similarities to the group of collagenosis. *Acta Med Scand.* 1964;**425** (suppl):14-8.
55. Judd PA, Finnegan P, Curran RC. Pulmonary sarcoidosis: a clinicopathologic study. *J Pathol.* 1975;**115**:191-8.
56. Cain H, Kraus B. Asteroid bodies: derivatives of the cytosphere. *Virchows Arch [Cell Pathol].* 1977;**26**:119-32.
57. Obel AL, Löfgren S. Pathogenesis of hyaline formation in sarcoidosis lymph nodes. *Acta Med Scand.* 1964;**425**(suppl):27-30.
58. DiBenedetto RJ, Ribaudo C. Bronchopulmonary sarcoidosis. *Am Rev Respir Dis.* 1966;**94**:952-5.
59. Scadding JG. The late stages of pulmonary sarcoidosis. *Postgrad Med J.* 1970;**46**:530-6.
60. Boros OL. Granulomatous inflammations. *Prog Allergy.* 1978;**24**:183-267.
61. Reynolds HY, Newball HH. Analysis of proteins and respiratory cells obtained from human lungs by bronchial lavage. *J Lab Clin Med.* 1974;**84**:559-73.
62. Reynolds HY, Fulmer JD Kazmierowski JA, Roberts WC, Frank MM, Crystal RG. Analysis of bronchoalveolar lavage fluid from patients with idiopathic pulmonary fibrosis and chronic hypersensitivity pneumonitis. *J Clin Invest.* 1977;**59**:165-75.
63. Weinberger SE, Kelman JA, Elson NA, et al. Bronchoalveolar lavage in interstitial lung disease. *Ann Intern Med.* 1978;**89**:459-66.
64. Hunninghake GW, Gadek JE, Szapiel SV, et al. The human alveolar macrophage. In: Harris CC, Trump BF, Stoner GD, eds. *Cultured Human Cells and Tissues in Bio-Medical Research.* New York: Academic Press; 1980. *(Methods and Perspectives in Cell Biology,* Vol. 1).
65. Hunninghake GW, Kawanami O, Ferrans VI, et al. Characterization of the inflammatory and immune effector cells in lung parenchyma of patients with interstitial lung disease. *Am Rev Respir Dis.* In press.
66. Yeager J, Williams MC, Beekman JF, Bayly TC, Beaman BL, Hawley RJ. Sarcoidosis: analysis of cells obtained by bronchial lavage. *Am Rev Respir Dis.* 1977;**116**:951-5.
67. Reynolds HY. The importance of lymphocytes in pulmonary health and disease. *Lung.* 1978;**155**:225-42.
68. Gee JB, Godel PT, Zorn SK, et al. Sarcoidosis and mononuclear

phagocytes. *Lung.* 1978;**155**:243-53.
69. Danel C, Arnoux A, Marsac J, et al. Cellular data from bronchoalveolar lavages in various interstitial diseases. *Bull Europ Physiopath Respir.* 1979;**15**:42P-43P.
70. Rossman MD, Daniele RP, Dauber JH. Bronchoalveolar lymphocytes in sarcoidosis. *Am Rev Respir Dis.* 1979;**119**:795.
71. Keogh B, Hunninghake G, Line B, et al. Therapeutic decisions in sarcoidosis: prospective evaluation of the effect of corticosteroids on lavage lymphocytes and [67] gallium scans. *Clin Res.* 1979;**27**:400A. Abstract.
72. Clot J, Andary M, Bonsequet J, Godart P, Michel FB. Lous populations lymphocytaires des iquides de lavage bronchoalveolaire. *Bull Europ Physiopath Respir.* 1979;**15**:27P-28P.
73. Barry BE, Crapo JD, Gehr P, Bachofen M, Weibel ER. Population characteristics of the cells in normal human lung. *Am Rev Respir Dis.* 1979;**119**:287A. Abstract.
74. Wybran JM, Carr C, Fudenbert HH. The human-rosette forming cell as a marker of a population of thymus-derived cells. *J Clin Invest.* 1972;**51**:2537-43.
75. Katoh AK, Charoensiri S. The formation of stable E-rosettes by human T-lymphocytes activated by phytohemagglutinin. *J Immunol.* 1977;**118**:2291-2.
76. Ferranrini M, Morretta L, Abile R, Durante ML. Receptors for IgG molecules on human lymphocytes forming spontaneous rosettes with sheep red cells. *Eur J Immunol.* 1975;**5**:70-2.
77. Krammer PH, Hudson C, Sprent J. Fc receptor, Ia-antigens, and immuno-globulin on normal and activated mouse T-lymphocytes. *J Exp Med.* 1975;**142**:1403-14.
78. Fridman WH, Fradelizi D, Guimezanes A, Plates C, Leclerc JC. The role of the Fc receptor (FcR) on thymus-derived lymphocytes. II. Presence of FcR on suppressor cells and direct involvement in suppression. *Eur J Immunol.* 1977;**8**:549-54.
79. Rossman MD, Dauber JH, Daniele RP. Elevation of stable (37°) E-rosettes in sarcoidosis. *Am Rev Respir Dis.* (suppl:73)1977:111.
80. Katz P, Haynes BF, Fauci AS. Alteration of T-lymphocyte subpopulations in sarcoidosis. *Clin Immunol Immunopathol.* 1978;**10**:350-4.
81. Hocking WG, Golde DW. The pulmonary-alveolar macrophage. *N Engl J Med.* 1979;**301**:580-7.
82. Blusse van Oud Alblas A, van Furth R. Origin, kinetics, and characteristics of pulmonary macrophages in the normal steady state. *J Exp Med.* 1979;**149**:1504-18.
83. Carr I. *The Macrophage.* London: Academic Press, Inc.; 1973:80-5.
84. Adams DO. The structure of mononuclear phagocytes differentiating *in vivo. Am J Pathol.* 1974;**76**:17-39.
85. Spector WG. The dynamics of granulomas and the significance of epithelioid cells. *Pathologie-Biologie.* 1975;**6**:437-9.
86. Black MM, Epstein WL. Formation of multinucleate giant cells in organized epithelioid cell granulomas. *Am J Pathol.* 1974;**74**:262-74.
87. Sutton JS, Weiss L. Transformation of monocytes in tissue culture into macrophages, epithelioid cells, and multinucleated giant cells: an electron microscope study. *J Cell Biol.* 1966;**28**:303-32.
88. Mariano M, Spector WG. The formation and properties of macrophage polykaryous (inflammatory giant cells). *J Pathol.* 1974;**113**:1-19.
89. Johnston RB Jr, Godzik CA, Cohn ZA. Increased superoxide anion production by immunologically activated and chemically elicited macrophages. *J Exp Med.* 1978;**148**:115-27.
90. Drath DB, Karnovsky ML, Huber GL. Hydroxyl radical formation in phagocytic cells of the rat. *Am J Physiol.* 1979;**46**:136-40.
91. Werb Z, Gordon S. Secretion of a specific collagenase by stimulated macrophages. *J Exp Med.* 1975;**142**:346-60.
92. Horowitz AL, Kelman JA, Crystal RG. Activation of alveolar macrophage collagenase by a neutral protease secreted by the same cell. *Nature.* 1976;**264**:772-4.
93. Janoff A, Rosenberg R, Gladston M. Elastase-like esteroprotease activity in human and rabbit alveolar macrophage granules. *Proc Soc Exp Biol Med.* 1971;**136**:1054-8.
94. Polverini PF, Cotran RS, Gimbrome MA, Unanue ER. Activated macrophages induce vascular proliferation. *Nature.* 1977;**269**:804-6.
95. Rosenthal AS, Lipsky PE, Shevach EM. Macrophage-lymphocyte interaction and antigen recognition. *Fed Proc.* 1975;**34**:1743-8.
96. Unanue ER. Secretory function of mononuclear phagocytes. *Am J Pathol.* 1976;**83**:396-417.
97. Evans R, Alexander P. Mechanisms of extracellular killing of nucleated mammalian cells by macrophages. In: Nelson DS, ed. *Immunobiology of the Macrophage.* New York: Academic Press; 1976:535-76.
98. Ward PA, Unanue ER, Goralnick SJ, Schreiner GF. Chemotaxis of rat lymphocytes. *J Immunol.* 1977;**119**:416-421.
99. Golde DW, Byers LD, Finley TN. Proliferative capacity of the human alveolar macrophage. *Nature.* 1974;**247**:373-5.
100. Adamson IYR, Bowden DH. Role of monocytes and interstitial cells in the generation of alveolar macrophages. *Fed Proc.* 1979;**38**:1205.
101. Boyden S. The chemotactic effect of mixtures of antibody and antigen on polymorphonuclear leukocytes. *J Exp Med.* 1962;**115**:453-66.
102. Kazmierowski JA, Gallin JI, Reynolds HY. Mechanisms for the inflammatory response in primate lungs: demonstration and partial characterization of an alveolar macrophage-derived chemotactic factor with preferential activity for polymorphonuclear leukocytes. *J Clin Invest.* 1977;**59**:273-81.
103. Hunninghake GW, Gallin JI, Fauci AS. Immunologic reactivity of the lung. The *in vivo* and *in vitro* generation of a neutrophil chemotactic factor by alveolar macrophages. *Am Rev Respir Dis.* 1978;**117**:15-23.
104. Hunninghake GW, Gadek JE, Crystal RG. Human alveolar macrophage chemotactic factor for neutrophils: stimuli and partial characterization. *J Clin Invest.* In press.
105. Merrill WW, Naegel GP, Matthay RA, Reynolds HY. Alveolar macrophage-derived chemotactic factor: kinetics of *in vitro* production and partial characterization. *J Clin Invest.* 1980;**65**:268-76.
106. Gadek JE, Hunninghake GW, Zimmerman RL, Crystal RG. Regulation of release of the alveolar macrophage-derived chemotactic factor. *Am Rev Respir Dis.* 1980;**121**:823-33.
107. Gallin JI, Quie PG. *Leukocyte Chemotaxis: Methods, Physiology, and Clinical Implications.* New York: Raven Press; 1978:1-429.
108. Ward PA, Remold HG, David JR. Leukotactic factor produced by sensitized lymphocytes. *Science.* 1969;**163**:1079-81.
109. Snyderman R, Altman LC, Hausman MS, et al. Human mononuclear leukocyte chemotaxis: a quantitative assay for humoral and cellular chemotactic factors. *J Immunol.* 1972;**108**:857-60.
110. Altman LC, Snyderman R, Oppenheim JJ, et al. A human mononuclear leukocyte chemotactic factor: characterization, specificity and kinetics of production by homologous leukocytes. *J Immunol.* 1973;**110**:801-10.
111. Kay AB, Stechschulte DJ, Austen KF. An eosinophilic leukocyte chemotactic factor of anaphylaxis. *J Exp Med.* 1971;**133**:602-19.
112. Zigmond SH, Hirsch JG. Leukocyte locomotion and chemotaxis: new methods for evaluation and demonstration of cell-derived chemotactic factor. *J Exp Med.* 1973;**137**:387-410.
113. Goetzl EJ, Woods JM, Gorman RR. Stimulation of human eosinophil and neutrophil polymorphonuclear leukocyte chemotaxis and random migration by 12-L-hydroxy-5,8,10,14-eicosatetraenoic acid. *J Clin Invest.* 1977;**59**:179-83.
114. Sobel JD, Gallin JI. Polymorphonuclear leukocyte and monocyte chemoattractants produced by human fibroblasts. *J Clin Invest.* 1979;**63**:609-18.
115. Kaplan AP, Goetzl EJ, Austen KF. The fibrinolytic pathway of human plasma. II. The generation of chemotactic activity by activation of plasminogen proactivator. *J Clin Invest.* 1973;**52**:2591-5.
116. Berenberg JL, Ward PA. Chemotactic factor inactivator in normal human serum. *J Clin Invest.* 1973;**52**:1200-6.
117. Goetzl EJ, Rocklin RE. Amplification of the activity of human leukocyte inhibitory factor (LIF) by the generatipn of a low molecular weight inhibitor of PMN leukocyte chemotaxis. *J Immuno.* 1978;**121**:891-6.
118. Till G, Ward PA. Two distinct chemotactic factor inactivators in human serum. *J Immunol.* 1975;**114**:843-7.
119. Rocklin RE. Products of activated lymphocytes: leukocyte inhibitory factor (LIF) distinct from migration inhibitory factor (MIF). *J Immunol.* 1974;**112**:1461-6.
120. Goetzl EJ. Plasma and cell-derived inhibitors of human neutrophil chemotaxis. *Ann NY Acad Sci.* 1975;**256**:210-21.
121. Wright DG, Gallin JI. Modulation of the inflammatory response by products released from human polymorphonuclear leukocytes during phagocytosis: generation and inactivation of the chemotactic factor C5a. *Inflammation.* 1975;**1**:23-39.
122. Cates KL, Ray CA Quie PG. Modified Boyden chamber method of measuring polymorphonuclear leukocyte chemotaxis. In: Gallin JI, Quie PG, eds. *Leukocyte Chemotaxis: Methods, Physiology, and Clinical Applications.* New York: Raven Press; 1978:67-72.
123. Altman LC. Chemotactic lymphokines. In: Gallin JI, Quie PG, eds. *Leukocyte Chemotaxis: Methods, Physiology, and Clinical Implications.* New York: Raven Press; 1978:267-88.
124. Gordon LI, Douglas SD, Kay NE, Yamada O, Osserman EF, Jacob HS. Modulation of neutrophil function by lysozyme: potential feedback system of inflammation. *J Clin Invest.* 1979;**64**:226-32.
125. Douglas SE, Doughaday CC, Schmidt ME, Siltzbach LE. Kinetics of monocyte receptor activity for immunoproteins in patients with sarcoidosis. *Ann NY Acad Sci.* 1976;**278**:190-6.
126. Douglas SE. Human monocyte spreading *in vitro*: inducers and effects on Fc and C3 receptors. *Cell Immunol.* 1976;**21**:344-9.
127. Himan LM, Stevens CA, Matthay RA, Reynolds HY, Gee JBL. Lysozyme and angiotensin convertase activity in human alveolar macrophages: the effects of cigarette smoking and pulmonary sarcoidosis.

Am Rev Respir Dis. 1978;**117**(Part 2):67. Abstract.
128. Shima K, Tamiya J, Tsuda T, Tokuomi H. Lysosomal enzyme activation of monocytes in sarcoid patients and activation factor in their sera. In: *Proceedings of the 8th International Conference on Sarcoidosis;* Cardiff, Wales, UK. 1978:9.
129. Friedland J, Setton C, Silverstein E. Induction of angiotensin converting enzyme in human monocytes in culture. *Biochem Biophys Res Comm.* 1979;**83**:843-9.
130. Silverstein E, Friedland J, Lyons HA, et al. Markedly elevated angiotensin converting enzyme in lymph nodes containing non-necrotizing granulomas in sarcoidosis. *Proc Nat Acad Sci USA.* 1976;**73**:2137-41.
131. Silverstein E, Friedland J, Lyons HA, et al. Elevation of angiotensin-converting enzyme in granulomatous lymph nodes and serum in sarcoidosis: clinical and possible pathogenic significance. *Ann NY Acad Sci.* 1976;**278**:498-513.
132. David JR, Remold HG. Macrophage activation by lymphocyte mediators and studies on the interaction of macrophages and lymphocytes. In: Nelson DS, ed. *Immunobiology of the Macrophage.* New York: Academic Press, 1976;401-27.
133. Gordon LI, Doublas SE, Kay NE, Osserman EF, Jacob HD. Modulation of neutrophil function by lysozyme: a macrophage secretory product. In: Williams WJ, Davies BH, eds. *Proceedings of the 8th International Conference on Sarcoidosis and Other Granulomatous Disease.* London: Alpha Omega Publishing, Ltd; 1980:76-83.
134. Maderazo EG, Ward PA, Woronick CL, Kubik J, DeGraff AC Jr. Leukotactic dysfunction in sarcoidosis. *Ann Intern Med.* 1976;**84**:414-9.
135. Campbell PB. Defective monocyte leukotaxis in sarcoidosis: possible relationship to a plasma factor. *Am Rev Respir Dis.* 1977;**116**:251-9.
136. Yoshida T, Siltzback LE, Masih N, Cohen S. Serum-migration inhibitory activity in patients with sarcoidosis. *Clin Immunol Immunopathol.* 1979;**13**:39-46.
137. Shima K, Ikeda S, Horiuchi S, Tokuomo H. Lysosomal enzyme activity of monocytes and activation factors in the sera of sarcoidosis patients. In: Williams WJ, Davies BH, eds. *Proceedings of the 8th International Conference on Sarcoidosis and Other Granulomatous Disease,* London: Alpha Omega Publishing, Ltd; 1980:89-98.
138. Semenzato G, Ciorani A, Colombatti M, Amadori G, Gasparotto G. Inhibitors of T-cell immune function in sarcoidosis. In: Williams WJ, Davies BH, eds. *Proceedings of the 8th International Conference on Sarcoidosis and Other Granulomatous Disease.* London: Alpha Omega Publishing, Ltd.; 1980:466-71.
139. Davies BH, Jones KP, Evans P, Jones-Williams W. Thymic lymphocyte responses in sarcoidosis: effect of sera and levamisole. In: Williams WJ, Davies BH, eds. *Proceedings of the 8th International Conference on Sarcoidosis and Other Granulomatous Disease.* London: Alpha Omega Publishing, Ltd.; 1980:477-84
140. Horsmanheimo A, Horsmanheimo M, Fudenberg HH, Siltzback LE, McKee KT. Kveins test reactivity with leukocyte migration in agarose and lymphocyte transformation tests. In: Williams WJ, Davies BH, eds. *Proceedings of the 8th International Conference on Sarcoidosis and Other Granulomatous Disease.* London: Alpha Omega Publishing, Ltd.; 1980:186-90.
141. Mangi RJ, Dwyer JM, Kantor FS. The effect of plasma upon lymphocyte responses *in vitro:* demonstration of a humoral inhibitor in patients with sarcoidosis. *Clin Exp Immunol.* 1974;**18**:519-28.
142. Drutz DJ, Cline MJ. Intermittent neutrophil-monocyte bactericidal defects in a patient with sarcoidosis. *Am Rev Respir Dis.* 1975;**112**:387-92.
143. Broom BC, Maclaurin BP. Sarcoidosis: correlation of delayed hypersensitivity, MLC reactivity and lymphocytotoxicity with disease activity. *Clin Exp Immunol.* 1973;**15**:355-64.
144. Friou GJ. Delayed cutaneous hypersensitivity in sarcoidosis. *J Clin Invest.* 1952;**31**:630.
145. Horsmanheimo M. Correlation of tuberculin-induced lymphocyte transformation with skin test reactivity and with clinical manifestations of sarcoidosis. *Cell Immunol.* 1974;**10**:329-37.
146. Kataria YP, LoBuglio AF, Bromberg PA. Sarcoid lymphocytes: spontaneous transformation and release of macrophage migration inhibition activity. *Am Rev Respir Dis.* 1976;**113**:315-23.
147. Selroos O, Niemisto M. Tuberculin sensitivity in active and cured sarcoidosis in Finland. In: Iwai K, Hosoda Y, eds. *Proceedings of the VI International Conference on Sarcoidosis,* Baltimore: University Park Press; 1974;248-52.
148. Sones M, Israel HL. Altered immunologic reactions in sarcoidosis. *Ann Intern Med.* 1954;**40**:260-8.
149. Veien NK, Hardt F, Bendixen G, et al. Immunological studies in sarcoidosis: a comparison of disease activity and various immunologic parameters. *Ann NY Acad Sci.* 1976;**278**:47-51.
150. Hoffbrand BI. Occurrence and significance of lymphopenia in sarcoidosis. *Am Rev Respir Dis.* 1968;**98**:107-10.
151. Sorensen SF, Hardt F, Veien NK. Estimation of lymphocyte subpopulations in the peripheral blood of patients with sarcoidosis. *Scand J Immunol.* 1976;**5**:1117-22.
152. Kalden JR, Peter HH, Lohmann E, Schedel J, Diehl V, Valke D. Estimation of T- and K-cell activity in the peripheral blood of sarcoidosis patients. *Ann NY Acad Sci.* 1976;**278**:52-68.
153. Hsu CCS, Wu SJY, Celic L, Weaver LJ, Solliday N. Increased proportion of active sheep erythrocyte rosette-forming lymphocytes and plasma rosette enhancement in sarcoidosis. *Am Rev Respir Dis.* 1979;**119**:383-9.
154. Goldstein RA, Janicki BW, Mirro J, Foellmer JW. Cell-mediated immune responses in sarcoidosis. *Am Rev Respir Dis.* 1978;**117**:55-62.
155. Siltzbach LE, Glade PR, Hirshant Y, Vieira LOBD, Celikoglu IS, Hirschhorn K. In vitro stimulation of peripheral lymphocytes in sarcoidosis. In: Levinsky L, Macholda F. *Fifth International Conference on Sarcoidosis.* Prague: University Karlova; 1971:217-20.
156. Daniele RP, McMillan LJ, Dauber JH, Rossman MD. Immune complexes in sarcoidosis: a correlation with activity and duration of disease. *Chest.* 1978;**74**:261-4.
157. Gupta RC, Kueppers F, DeRemee RA, et al. Pulmonary and extrapulmonary sarcoidosis in relation to circulating immune complexes: a quantification of immune complexes by two radioimmunoassays. *Am Rev Respir Dis.* 1977;**116**:261-6.
158. Hedfors E, Norberg R. Evidence for circulating immune complexes in sarcoidosis. *Clin Exp Immunol.* 1974;**16**:493-6.
159. Verrier-Jones J, Cumming RH, Asplin CM. Evidence for circulating immune complexes in erythema nodosum and early sarcoidosis. *Ann NY Acad Sci.* 1976;**278**:212-9.
160. Kueppers F, DeRemee RE. Search for a specific antibody in sera from patients with sarcoidosis. *Ann NY Acad Sci.* 1976;**278**:220-4.
161. Daniele RP, Rowlands DT. Antibodies to T cells in sarcoidosis. *Ann NY Acad Sci.* 1976;**278**:88-100.
162. Klockars M, Selroos O. Immunohistochemical demonstration of lysozyme in the lymph nodes and Kveim reaction papules in sarcoidosis. *Acta Pathol Microbiol Scand.* 1977;**85A**:169-73.
163. Pascual RS, Gee JBL, Finch SC. Usefulness of serum lysozyme measurement in diagnosis and evaluation of sarcoidosis. *N Engl J Med.* 1973;**289**:1074-6.
164. Selroos O, Klockars M. Serum lysozyme in sarcoidosis. Evaluation of its usefulness in determination of disease activity. *Scand J Respir Dis.* 1977;**58**:110-6.
165. Silverstein E, Friedland J, Ackerman T. Elevation of granulomatous lymph node and serum lysozyme in sarcoidosis and correlation with angiotensin-converting enzyme. *Am J Clin Pathol.* 1977;**68**:219-24.
166. Siltzback LE, Krakoff L, Dorph D, Tierstein AS. Elevated levels of serum angiotensin-converting enzyme (ACE) and lysozyme (L) levels in sarcoidosis. In: Williams WJ, Davies BH, eds. *Proceedings of the 8th International Conference on Sarcoidosis and Other Granulomatous Disease.* London: Alpha Omega Publishing, Ltd.; 1980:298-302.
167. Ashutosh K, Keighley JFH. Diagnostic value of serum angiotensin converting enzyme activity in lung disease. *Thorax.* 1976;**31**:552-7.
168. Fanburg BL, Schoenberger MD, Bachus B, Snider GL. Elevated serum angiotensin I converting enzyme in sarcoidosis. *Am Rev Respir Dis.* 1976;**114**:525-8.
169. Ferlitsch A, Kohout J, Kummer F, Legenstein E, Muller MM. Angiotensin converting enzyme in the diagnosis of sarcoidosis. In: Williams WJ, Davies BH, eds. *Proceedings of the 8th International Conference on Sarcoidosis and Other Granulomatous Disease.* London: Alpha Omega Publishing, Ltd.; 1980:22.
170. Lieberman J. Elevation of serum angiotensin-converting-enzyme (ACE) level in sarcoidosis. *Am J Med.* 1975;**59**:365-72.
171. Lieberman J. The specificity and nature of serum angiotensin-converting-enzyme (serum ACE) elevations in sarcoidosis. *Ann NY Acad Sci.* 1976;**278**:488-97.
172. Lieberman J, Kaneshiro W, Weisser K, et al. Update on serum ACE: angiotensin converting enzyme assays for diagnosis and therapeutic evaluation in sarcoidosis. In: Williams WJ, Davies BH, eds. *Proceedings of the 8th International Conference on Sarcoidosis and Other Granulomatous Disease.* London: Alpha Omega Publishing, Ltd.; 1980:320-7.
173. Rohrbach MS, DeReme RA. Serum angiotensin converting enzyme activity in sarcoidosis as measured by a simple radiochemical assay. *Am Rev Respir Dis.* 1979;**119**:761-7.
174. Sandron D, Lecossier D, Moreun F, Basset G, Battesti JP. Comparison between two methods of determining serum angiotensin converting enzyme in sarcoidosis and other pulmonary diseases. In: Williams WJ, Davies BH, eds. *Proceedings of the 8th International Conference on Sarcoidosis and Other Granulomatous Disease.* London: Alpha Omega Publishing, Ltd.; 1980; 317-9.
175. Abboy R, Kanada DJ, Sharma OP. Serum angiotensin converting

enzyme in sarcoidosis. In: WILLIAMS WJ, DAVIES BH, eds. *Proceedings of the 8th International Conference on Sarcoidosis and Other Granulomatous Disease.* London: Alpha Omega Publishing; 1980:273-6.

176. SIMONOWITZ LJ, SOLLIDAY N, CELIC L, CUGELL E. Serial measurements of angiotensin converting enzyme and diffusing capacity in sarcoidosis. *Am Rev Respir Dis.* 1977;**115**(suppl):164. Abstract.
177. STUDDY P, BIRD R, GERAINT JD, SHERBERB S. Serum angiotensin converting enzyme (SACE) in sarcoidosis and other granulomatous disorders. In: WILLIAMS WJ, DAVIES BH, eds. *Proceedings of the 8th International Conference on Sarcoidosis and Other Granulomatous Disease.* London: Alpha Omega Publishing, Ltd.; 1980:259-65.
178. UEDA E, HISHIMURAK, HAWADA K, et al. Serum angiotensin-converting enzyme activity in patients with sarcoidosis. *Jpn J Thorac Dis.* 1976;**14**:736-42.
179. NELSON DS. *Immunobiology of the Macrophage.* New York: Academic Press; 1976.
180. PASCUAL RS, PERILLE PE, GEE JBL, FINCH SC. Serum and urine lysozyme in sarcoidosis. In: OSSERMAN E, CENFIELD R, BEYCHOK S, eds. *Lysozyme.* New York: Academic Press; 1974:391.
181. NG KKF, VANE JR. Fate of angiotensin I in the circulation. *Nature (London).* 1968;**218**:144-50.
182. RENZI G, DUTTON RE. Pulmonary function in diffuse sarcoidosis. *Respiration.* 1973;**31**:124-31.
183. JAMES DG, CARSTAIRS LS, TROWELL J, SHARMA OP. Treatment of sarcoidosis: report of a controlled therapeutic trial. *Lancet.* 1967;**2**:526-8.
184. KIRKS DR, MCCORMICK VD, GREENSPAN RH. Pulmonary sarcoidosis: roentgenologic analysis of 150 patients. *Am J Roentgenol Radium Therap Nucl Med.* 1973;**117**:777-8.
185. JAMES DG. Diagnosis and treatment of sarcoidosis. *Br Med J.* 1956;**2**:900-04.
186. JAMES DG, NEVILLE E, SILTZBACH LE, et al. A worldwide view of sarcoidosis. *Ann NY Acad Sci.* 1976;**278**:321-34.
187. DEREMEE RA, ANDERSEN HA. Sarcoidosis: a correlation of dyspnea with roentgenographic stage and pulmonary function changes. *Mayo Clin Proc.* 1974;**49**:742-5.
188. FREUNDLICH IM, LIBSHITZ HI, GLASSMAN LM, ISRAEL HL. Sarcoidosis: typical and atypical thoracic manifestations and complications. *Clin Radiol.* 1970;**21**:376-83.
189. FRASER RG, PARE JAP. *Diagnosis of Diseases of the Chest.* Philadelphia: W.B. Saunders; 1979:1659-90.
190. FELSON B. *Chest Roentgenology.* Philadelphia: W.B. Saunders; 1973:302.
191. RABINOWITZ JG, ULREICH S, SORIANO C. The usual unusual manifestations of sarcoidosis and the "hilar haze"—a new diagnostic aid. *Am J Roentgenol Rad Therap Nucl Med.* 1974;**120**:821-39.
192. SHIGEMATSU N, EMORI K, MATSUBA K, HARADA S, TAKAHAHI T. Clinico-pathologic characteristics of pulmonary acinar sarcoidosis. *Chest.* 1978;**73**:186-8.
193. FELSON B. Uncommon roentgen patterns of pulmonary sarcoidosis. *Dis Chest.* 1958;**34**:357-67.
194. SHARMA OP, HEWLETT R, GORDONSON J. Nodular sarcoidosis: an unusual radiographic appearance. *Chest.* 1973;**64**:189-92.
195. KIRKS DR, MCCORMICK VD, GREENSPAN RH. Pulmonary sarcoidosis: roentgenologic analysis of 150 patients. *Am J Roentgenol.* 1973;**117**:777-86.
196. YOUNG RC, TITUS-DILLON PY, SCHNEIDER ML, SHELTON TG, HACKNEY RL, HARDEN KA. Sarcoidosis in Washington, D.C.: clinical observations in 105 black patients. In: LEVINSKY DL, MACHOLDA F, eds. *Fifth International Conference on Sarcoidosis.* Prague: Universita Karlova; 1971:513-20.
197. ROSEN Y, AMOROSA JK, MOON S, COHEN J, LYONS HA. Occurrence of lung granulomas in patients with stage I sarcoidosis. *Am J Roentgenol.* 1977;**129**:1083-85.
198. EPLER GR, MCLOUD TC, GAENSLER ER, MICKUS JP, CARRINGTON CB. Normal chest roentgenograms in chronic diffuse infiltrative lung disease. *N Engl J Med.* 1978;**298**:934-9.
199. MCCORT JJ, PARE JAP. Pulmonary fibrosis and cor pulmonale in sarcoidosis. *Radiology.* 1954;**62**:496-504.
200. SCADDING JG. Prognosis of intrathoracic sarcoidosis. *Br Med J.* 1961;**2**:1165-72.
201. MIKHAIL JR, DRURY RA, MITCHELL DN. Evaluation of the clinical and histological features of paratracheal and hilar gland enlargement. *Postgrad Med J.* 1970;**46**:515-8.
202. BOUSHY SF, KURTZMAN RS, MARTIN ND, LEWIS BM. The course of pulmonary function in sarcoidosis. *Ann Intern Med.* 1965;**62**:939-55.
203. BERG GR. Pulmonary function in sarcoidosis. *N Engl J Med.* 1968;**278**:1019. Letter.
204. O'BRIEN LE, FORSMAN PJ, WILTSE HE. Early onset sarcoidosis with pulmonary function abnormalities. *Chest.* 1974;**65**:472-4.
205. RENZI G, DUTTON RE. Pulmonary function in diffuse sarcoidosis. *Respiration.* 1974;**31**:124-36.
206. COLP C, PARK SS, WILLIAMS MH JR. Pulmonary function follow-up to 120 patients with sarcoidosis. *Ann NY Acad Sci.* 1976;**278**:301-07.
207. MILLER A, CHUANG M, TEIRSTEIN AS, SILTZBACH LE. Pulmonary function in stage I and II pulmonary sarcoidosis. *Ann NY Acad Sci.* 1976;**278**:292-300.
208. HAMER NA. Changes in the components of the diffusing capacity in pulmonary sarcoidosis. *Thorax.* 1963;**18**:275-87.
209. SAUMON G, GEORGES R, LOISEAU A, TURIAF J. Membrane diffusing capacity and pulmonary capillary blood volume in pulmonary sarcoidosis. *Ann NY Acad Sci.* 1976;**278**:284-91.
210. SELLERS RD, SIEBENS AA. The effects of sarcoidosis on pulmonary function with particular reference to changes in pulmonary compliance. *Am Rev Respir Dis.* 1965;**91**:660-4.
211. TING GY, WILLIAMS MH JR. Mechanics of breathing in sarcoidosis of the lung. *JAMA.* 1965;**192**:619-24.
212. HARDEN KA, YOUNG RC JR, CARR C, LAUREY JR. Oxygen cost of breathing. II. Studies in patients with sarcoidosis. *Am Rev Respir Dis.* 1968;**97**:1127-30.
213. SNIDER GL, DOCTOR LR. The mechanics of ventilation in sarcoidosis. *Am Rev Respir Dis.* 1964;**89**:897-908.
214. TABIRI G, ARNDT H, BEHREND H, DOMBROWSKI H. Lung volumes, compliance and diffusing capacity in advanced pulmonary sarcoidosis. In: LEVINSKY DL, MACHOLDA F, eds. *Fifth International Conference on Sarcoidosis.* Prague: Universita Karlova; 1971:442-6.
215. YOUNG RL, HARKLEROAD CE, LORDON RE, WEG JG. Pulmonary sarcoidosis: a prospective evaluation of glucocorticoid therapy. *Ann Intern Med.* 1970;**73**:207-12.
216. KANEKO K, SHARMA OP. Airway obstruction in pulmonary sarcoidosis. *Bull Eur Physiopathol Respir.* 1977;**13**:231-40.
217. RIZZATO G, BRAMBILLA I, BERTOLI L, CONTI F, MERLIN R, MANTARO O. Impaired airway function and pulmonary hemodynamics in sarcoidosis. In: WILLIAMS WJ, DAVIES BH, eds. *Proceedings of the 8th International Conference on Sarcoidosis and Other Granulomatous Disease.* London: Alpha Omega Publishing, Ltd.; 1980:349-60.
218. SAHETYA GK, COVY WB, FACEN HK, HASSAN S, KUMAR B, YOUNG RC. Pulmonary sarcoidosis: a significant cause of chronic airway obstruction. In: WILLIAMS WJ, DAVIES, BH, eds. *Proceedings of the 8th International Conference on Sarcoidosis and Other Granulomatous Disease.* London: Alpha Omega Publishing, Ltd.; 1980:361-7.
219. MILLER A, TEIRSTEIN AS, JACKLER I, CHUANG M, SILTZBACH LE. Airway function in chronic pulmonary sarcoidosis with fibrosis. *Am Rev Respir Dis.* 1974;**109**:179-89.
220. TAMMELING GJ, DE VRIES K, SLUITER HJ, et al. Obstructive lung disease in pulmonary sarcoidosis. *Acta Med Scand.* 1964;**176**(suppl):275-77.
221. LEVINSON RS, METZGER LF, STANLEY NN, et al. Airway function in sarcoidosis. *Am J Med.* 1977;**62**:51-9.
222. RADWAN L, GREBSKA E, KOZIOROWSKI A. Small airway function in pulmonary sarcoidosis. *Scand J Respir Dis.* 1978;**59**:37-43.
223. SHARMA OP. Airway obstruction in sarcoidosis. *Chest.* 1978;**73**:6-7. Editorial.
224. BATES DV, MACKLEM PT, CHRISTIE RV. Pulmonary sarcoidosis, In: *Respiratory Function in Disease.* Philadelphia: W.B. Saunders Co.; 1971:287-9.
225. STANECK V, WIDIMSKY J, NAVRATIL M, DAUM S, LEVINSKY L. The pulmonary gas exchange during exercise in patients with pulmonary fibrosis. *Scand J Respir Dis.* 1967;**48**:11-2.
226. SEARS MR. Pulmonary gas transfer and alveolar-oxygen differences in sarcoidosis. In: WILLIAMS WJ, DAVIES BH, eds. *Proceedings of the 8th International Conference on Sarcoidosis and Other Granulomatous Disease.* London: Alpha Omega Publishing, Ltd.; 1980:343-8.
227. COLP C. Sarcoidosis: course and treatment. *Med Clin N Am.* 1977;**61**:1267-78.
228. YOUNG RC JR, CARR C, SHELTON TG, et al. Sarcoidosis: relationship between changes in lung structure and function. *Am Rev Respir Dis.* 1967;**95**:224-38.
229. YOUNG RL, LORDON RE, KRUMHOLZ RA, HARKLEROAD LE, BRANAM GE, WEG JG. Pulmonary sarcoidosis. I. Pathophysiologic correlations. *Am Rev Respir Dis.* 1968;**97**:997-1008.
230. EDWARDS CL, HAYES RL. Tumor scanning with ^{67}Ga citrate. *J Nucl Med.* 1969;**10**:103-5.
231. LAVENDER PJ, LOWE J, BARKER JR, BURN JI, CHAUDHRI MA. Gallium-67 citrate scanning in neoplastic and inflammatory lesions. *Br J Radiol.* 1971;**44**:361-6.
232. KANNO I. Diagnostic evaluation of ^{67}Ga scanning of lung cancer and other diseases. *Radiology.* 1971;**101**:355-62.
233. HISASI T, NAKAYAMA Y. Clinical evaluation of ^{67}Ga citrate scanning. *J Nucl Med.* 1972;**13**:196-201.
234. VAN DER SCHOOT JB, GROEN AS, DE JONS J. Gallium-67 scintigraphy in lung diseases. *Thorax.* 1972;**27**:543-6.
235. TEATES CD, BRAY ST, WILLIAMSON BR. Tumor detection with ^{67}Ga citrate: a literature survey (1970-1978). *Clin Nucl Med.* 1978;**3**:456-60.
236. DISE-PETERSON H, HECKSCHER T, HERTZ M. ^{67}Ga-scintigraphy in

nonmalignant lung diseases. *Scand J Respir Dis.* 1972;**53**:314-31.

237. Littenberg RL, Taketa RM, Alazraki NP, Halpern SE, Ashburn WL. Gallium-67 for localization of septic lesions. *Ann Intern Med.* 1973;**79**:403-6.
238. Israel HL, Atkinson GW. Sarcoidosis: basics of respiratory disease. *Am Thoracic Soc.* 1978;**7**:1-6.
239. Silberstein EB. Gallium detection of inflammation. *Ann Intern Med.* 1974;**80**:774. Letter.
240. Teates CD, Hunger JG. Gallium scanning as a screening test for inflammatory lesions. *Radiology.* 1975;**116**:383-7.
241. Kumar B, Coleman RE, Alderson PO. Gallium citrate Ga-67 imaging in patients with suspected inflammatory processes. *Arch Surg.* 1975;**110**:1237-42.
242. Siemsen JK, Grebe SF, Sargent EN, Wentz D. Gallium-67 scintigraphy of pulmonary diseases as a complement to radiography. *Radiology.* 1976;**118**:371-5.
243. Vallieres BJ, Johnston GS, Jones AE, Line BR. Gallium-67 citrate scintigraphy: II. Clinical aspects. *Union Med Can.* 1977;**106**:1382-91.
244. Staab EV, McCartney WH. Role of gallium-67 in inflammatory disease. *Semin Nucl Med.* 1978;**8**:219-34.
245. Myerson PJ, Myerson DA, Spencer RP. Anatomic correlations in radiogallium imaging of the peritoneum and retroperitoneum. *Semin Nucl Med.* 1979;**9**:66-70.
246. Lanshammer H, Glaubitt G, Grebe SF, et al. Gallium-67 for tumor scanning. *J Nucl Med.* 1972;**13**:25-30.
247. Nelson B, Hayes RL, Edwards CL, et al. Distribution of gallium in human tissues after intravenous administration. *J Nucl Med.* 1972;**13**:92-100.
248. Larson SM, Milder MS, Johnston GS. Interpretation of the ^{67}Ga photoscan. *J Nucl Med.* 1973;**14**:208-14.
249. Line BR, Fulmer JD, Reynolds HY, et al. Gallium-67 citrate scanning in the staging of idiopathic pulmonary fibrosis: correlation with physiologic and morphologic features and bronchoalveolar lavage. *Am Rev Respir Dis.* 1978;**118**:355-65.
250. Siemsen JK, Grebe SF, Waxman AD. The use of gallium-67 in pulmonary disorders. *Semin Nucl Med.* 1978;**8**:235-49.
251. Heshiki A, Schatz SL, McKusick KA, Bowersox DW, Soin JS, Wagner HN. Gallium-67 citrate scanning in patients with pulmonary sarcoidosis. *Am J Roentgenol Radium Ther Nucl Med.* 1974;**122**:744-9.
252. Mertz T, Malmud L, McKusick KA, Wagner HN. Mechanisms of ^{67}Ga association with lymphocytes. *Cancer Res.* 1974;**34**:2495-9.
253. Niden AH, Mishkin FS, Khurana ML. ^{67}Gallium citrate lung scans in interstitial lung disease. *Chest.* 1976;**69**:266-8.
254. Stone DJ, Schwartz A, Feltman JA, Lovelock FJ. Pulmonary function in sarcoidosis: results with cortisone therapy. *Am J Med.* 1953;**15**:468-78.
255. Israel HL, Sones M, Harrell D. Cortisone treatment of sarcoidosis: experience with thirty-six cases. *JAMA.* 1954;**156**:461-8.
256. Smellie H, Apthorp GH, Marshall R. The effect of corticosteroid treatment on pulmonary function in sarcoidosis. *Thorax.* 1960;**16**:87-90.
257. Sharma OP, Colp C, Williams MH. Course of pulmonary sarcoidosis with and without corticosteroid therapy as determined by pulmonary function studies. *Am J Med.* 1966;**41**:541-51.
258. Siltzbach LE. Sarcoidosis: clinical features and management. *Med Clin N Am.* 1967;**51**:483-502.
259. American Thoracic Society Medical Section of the National Tuberculosis and Respiratory Disease Association: Treatment of sarcoidosis. *Am Rev Respir Dis.* 1971;**103**:433-4.
260. Israel HL, Fouts DW, Beggs RA. A controlled trial of prednisone treatment of sarcoidosis. *Am Rev Respir Dis.* 1973;**107**:609-14.
261. Johns CJ, Zachary JB, Ball WC. A ten-year study of corticosteroid treatment of pulmonary sarcoidosis. *Hopkins Med J.* 1974;**134**:271-83.
262. Hedfors E. Influence of steroid treatment on lymphocyte response in sarcoidosis. *Clin Immunol Immunopathol.* 1975;**4**:96-100.
263. Balow JE, Hurley DL, Fauci AS. Immuno-suppressive effects of glucocorticoids: differential effects of acute vs. chronic administration on cell-mediated immunity. *J Immunol.* 1975;**114**:1072-6.
264. Fauci AS, Dale DC, Balow JE. Glucocorticosteroid therapy: mechanisms of action and clinical considerations. *Ann Intern Med.* 1976;**84**:304-15.
265. Rosenau W, Moon HD. The inhibitory effect of hydrocortisone on lysis of homologous cells by lymphocytes in vitro. *J Immunol.* 1962;**89**:422-6.
266. Stavey L, Cohen IR, Feldman M. The effect of hydrocortisone on lymphocyte-mediated cytolysis. *Cell Immunol.* 1973;**7**:302-12.
267. Fauci AS. Corticosteroids and circulating lymphocytes. *Transplant Proc.* 1975;**7**:37-40.
268. Haynes BF, Fauci AS. The differential effect of in vivo hydrocortisone on the kinetics of subpopulations of human peripheral blood thymus-derived lymphocytes. *J Clin Invest.* 1978;**61**:703-7.
269. Balow JE, Rosenthal AS. Glucocorticoid suppression of macrophage migration inhibitory factor. *J Exp Med.* 1973;**137**:1031-41.
270. Crystal RG, Fulmer JD, Baum B, et al. Cells, collagen and idiopathic pulmonary fibrosis. *Lung.* 1978;**155**:199-224.
271. Vracko R. Significance of basal lamina for regeneration of injured lung. *Virchows Arch [Pathol Anat].* 1972;**355**:264-74.
272. British Tuberculosis Association: Chloroquine in the treatment of sarcoidosis. *Tubercle.* 1967;**48**:257-72.
273. Breyne H. Experiences with immunological therapy of sarcoidosis over 13 years. *Z Erkrank Atm Org.* 1977;**149**:160-3.
274. Wandett-Freerksen E. Aldactone in the treatment of sarcoidosis of the lungs. *Z Erkrank Atm Org.* 1977;**149**:156-9.
275. Rosof BM. Allopurinol for sarcoid. *N Engl J Med.* 1964;**294**:447. Letter.
276. Rosenthal M, Trabert U, Müller W, Müller S, Wurm K. Levamisole in sarcoidosis. *N Engl J Med.* 1974;**294**:112-3.
277. Hedfors E. Possible role for anticoagulant treatment in sarcoidosis. *Mt Sinai J Med.* 1977;**44**:745-7.
278. Geraint-James D, Carstairs LS, Trowell J, Sharma OP. Treatment of sarcoidosis: report of a controlled therapeutic trial. *Lancet.* 1967:526-8.
279. Israel HL. Effects of chlorambucil and methotrexate in sarcoidosis. In: Levinsky L, Mackolda F, eds. *Fifth International Conference on Sarcoidosis.* Prague: Universita Karlova; 1971:632-4.
280. Sharma O, Hughes DTD, Geraint-James D, Naish P. Immunosuppressive therapy with azathioprine in sarcoidosis. In: Levinsky L, Macholda F, eds. *Fifth International Conference on Sarcoidosis.* Prague: Universita Karlova; 1971:635-7.

Heart Transplantation for Undiagnosed Cardiac Sarcoidosis

Alan S. Donsky, MD, Juan Escobar, MD, John Capehart, MD, and William C. Roberts, MD

Heart transplantation (HT) for cardiac sarcoidosis is rare. Only 6 patients having HT for cardiac sarcoidosis have been previously reported[1–4] (Table 1). In 2 of them, the diagnosis of cardiac sarcoidosis was not known at the time of HT. In this report, we describe a patient who underwent HT for presumed idiopathic dilated cardiomyopathy (IDC), but on examination, the explanted heart was found to have extensive cardiac sarcoidosis.

• • •

A 53-year-old white man was well until age 41 when he developed exertional dyspnea and palpitations. Examination at that time disclosed a blood pressure of 110/70 mm Hg, and a heart rate of 60 beats/min. There was no jugular venous distention or peripheral edema present but an S3 and S4 gallop was heard on auscultation. An electrocardiogram showed normal sinus rhythm with a prolonged PR interval (240 ms) and complete left bundle branch block (QRS duration 160 ms) (Figure 1). Total 12-lead QRS voltage = 110 mm (10 mm = 1 mV). An echocardiogram disclosed dilation of the right and left ventricles (left ventricular end-diastolic diameter = 60 mm, and peak systolic diameter = 38 mm) and global hypokinesia with an ejection fraction of 25%. Exercise thallium stress tests showed no resting or exercise-induced perfusion defects. IDC was diagnosed. Two years later he developed symptomatic sustained ventricular tachycardia requiring electrical cardioversion and implantation of an automatic implantable cardioverter-defibrillator.

Despite optimal medical management, his heart failure progressed. A repeat echocardiogram at age 49 showed that his ejection fraction had fallen to 15%. Right-sided cardiac catheterization showed a cardiac index of 1.5 L/min/m^2, a pulmonary artery pressure of 43/24 mm Hg, and a mean pulmonary wedge pressure of 26 mm Hg. At age 53 (September 1999) he underwent orthotopic HT.

Examination of the native (recipient) heart showed extensive focal scarring of the right ventricular wall, the cephalad portion of the ventricular septum, and the lateral, anterior, and posterior left ventricular walls (Figure 2). The heart weighed 510 g. All epicardial coronary arteries were widely patent. Microscopic sections disclosed numerous multinucleated giant cells and lymphocytes, mainly within the scarred areas (Figure 3).

As of May 1, 2002, the patient is asymptomatic. None of his posttransplant biopsy specimens have shown recurrence of sarcoid.

• • •

Sarcoidosis is an idiopathic, systemic, granulomatous disease that can affect any organ system, although the lymph nodes and lungs are most often affected. Cardiac involvement was first described by Bernstein et al[5] in 1929. Not much was known about cardiac sarcoidosis until Gozo et al[6] reviewed 70 autopsy cases of patients who died from primary cardiac sarcoidosis. The average age of death was 40 years. The most common clinical manifestations were conduction disturbances, ventricular arrhythmias, and congestive heart failure. In 1977, Roberts and colleagues[7] reported on 113 necropsy patients with cardiac sarcoidosis. They found that sarcoid granulomas and scars most often involved the left ventricular free wall and the cephalad portion of the ventricular septum. Furthermore, they observed that patients in whom sarcoidosis had caused cardiac dysfunction had little or no clinical evidence of dysfunction in any other organ system. The incidence of cardiac involvement in patients with pulmonary sarcoidosis was studied by Silverman and colleagues[8] in 1978. They reviewed 84 autopsy cases of pulmonary sarcoidosis in the files of The Johns Hopkins Hospital and found grossly visible myocardial sarcoid lesions in only 4 patients (5%), although another 19 (23%) had noncaseating granulomas in microscopic sections of myocardium. Our patient had severe cardiac dysfunction caused by sarcoidosis without extracardiac symptoms.

Differentiating cardiac sarcoidosis from IDC can be difficult. Yazaki et al[9] retrospectively compared 15 patients having cardiac sarcoidosis and left ventricular systolic dysfunction (ejection fraction <40% and left ventricular end-diastolic diameter >55 mm) with 30 patients with IDC. The sarcoidosis group had a statistically significant higher frequency of complete heart block (67% vs 0%), right bundle branch block (57% vs 17%), and abnormal left ventricular wall thickness (73% vs 17%). Flemming[10] found that patients with cardiac sarcoidosis who developed complete heart block developed it at a much younger age than those with idiopathic heart block, so that complete heart block in a young patient may be a clue to undiagnosed cardiac sarcoidosis.

Endomyocardial biopsy can confirm the diagnosis of cardiac sarcoidosis by the presence of noncaseating epithelioid granulomas.

From the Departments of Internal Medicine (Division of Cardiology) and Cardiothoracic Surgery and Pathology, the Heart and Vascular Institute, Baylor University Medical Center, Dallas, Texas. Dr. Roberts' address is: Baylor Heart and Vascular Institute, Baylor University Medical Center, 3600 Gaston Avenue, Dallas, Texas 75246. Manuscript received January 9, 2002; revised manuscript received and accepted February 25, 2002.

TABLE 1 Clinical and Morphologic Cardiac Data in Previously Reported Patients Having Cardiac Transplantation for Cardiac Sarcoidosis

Case	First Author	Publication Year	Age at HT (yrs)	Race	Sex	Pre-HT Dx of Sarcoid	Reason for HT	Died (months Lived after HT)	Occurrence of Sarcoid After HT	Native Heart Weight (g)	Location of Granulomas						Dilated		BBB	CHB	VT	Prolonged PR Interval
											RA	RV	LA	LV	AS	VS	RV	LV				
1	Gokel	1985	37	-	M	+ (Bx)	-	+ (8)	-	-	-	-	-	-	-	-	-	-	-	-	-	-
2	Valantine	1987	46	W	M	0	VT	+ (42)	0 (A)	630	-	+	-	+	-	+	0	0	+ (R)	0	+	+
3	Valantine	1987	47	B	M	+ (Bx)	CHF	0 (16+)	0 (Bx)	420	"Widespread"						0	+	0	0	+	+
4	Valantine	1987	51	W	F	0 (Bx)	CHF	0 (20+)	0 (Bx)	400	-	0	-	+	-	+	-	-	+ (R)	0	0	+
5	Oni	1992	34	-	M	+ (Bx)	CHF	0 (13+)	+ (Bx)	-	-	-	-	-	-	-	+	+	0	0	+	0
6	Ankersmi	2001	30	-	M	+ (Bx)	CHF	0 (1+)	-	-	-	-	-	-	-	-	+	+	0	0	+	0

A = autopsy; AS = atrial septum; B = black; BBB = bundle branch block; Bx = biopsy; CHB = complete heart block; CHF = congestive heart failure; Dx = diagnosis; LA = left atrium; LV = left ventricle; R = right; RA = right atrium; RV = right ventricle; VS = ventricular septum; VT = ventricular tachycardia; W = white; - = no information available.

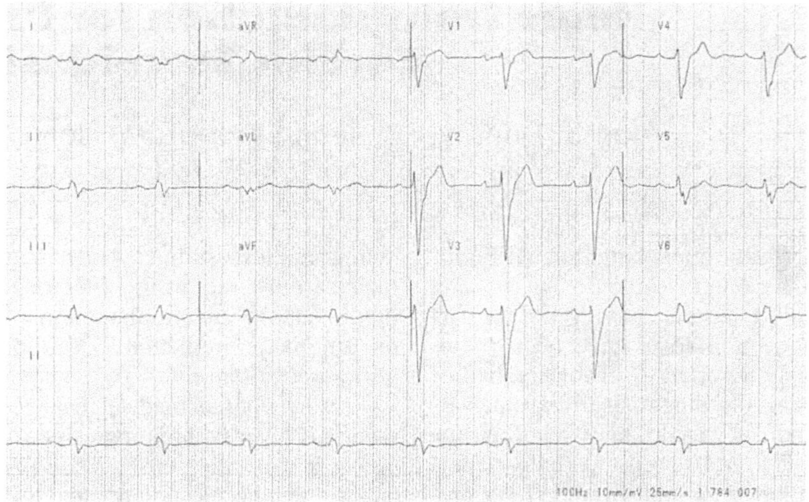

FIGURE 1. Electrocardiogram in the patient described. The electrocardiogram shows sinus rhythm, prolonged PR interval (0.24 second), and complete left bundle branch block (QRS duration = 0.16 second).

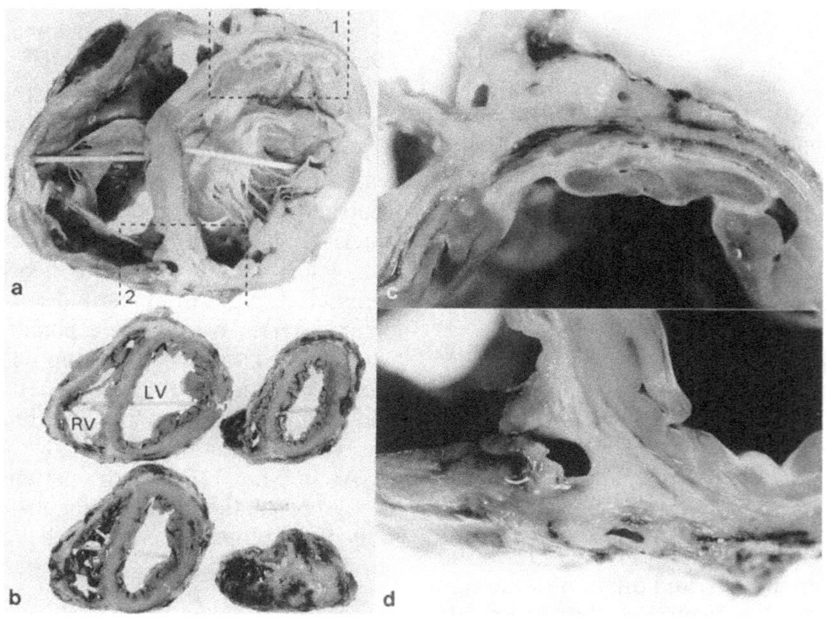

FIGURE 2. The heart in the patient described. *a,* view of the base of the heart after excision of the more apical portion of the right and left ventricles. Both ventricular cavities are considerably dilated. The area 1 *(shown in box with broken line)* is magnified in *c.* The left ventricular free wall and ventricular septum and a portion of anterior wall of the right ventricle (RV) in its outflow track is severely scarred and the wall is thinned. A close-up of area 2 is shown in *d.* Again the posterior portion of the left ventricular free wall, the right ventricular aspect of the ventricular septum, and a portion of the right ventricular free wall adjacent to the septum are severely scarred. *b,* transverse views of the right and left ventricular cavities and walls in the more apical portions of the heart. The ventricular cavities again are quite dilated. LV = left ventricle.

Its diagnostic yield is difficult to determine because the gold standard for the diagnosis of cardiac sarcoidosis is autopsy. Several studies, however, have reported on its diagnostic yield in patients with suspected cardiac sarcoidosis. In 1 study of 26 patients in whom cardiac sarcoidosis was "strongly suspected," only 5 (19%) had noncaseating granulomas on biopsy.[11] In another study involving 8 patients, only 2 had noncaseating granulomas.[12] This low yield is likely due to the patchy nature of the granulomas and their predilection for the

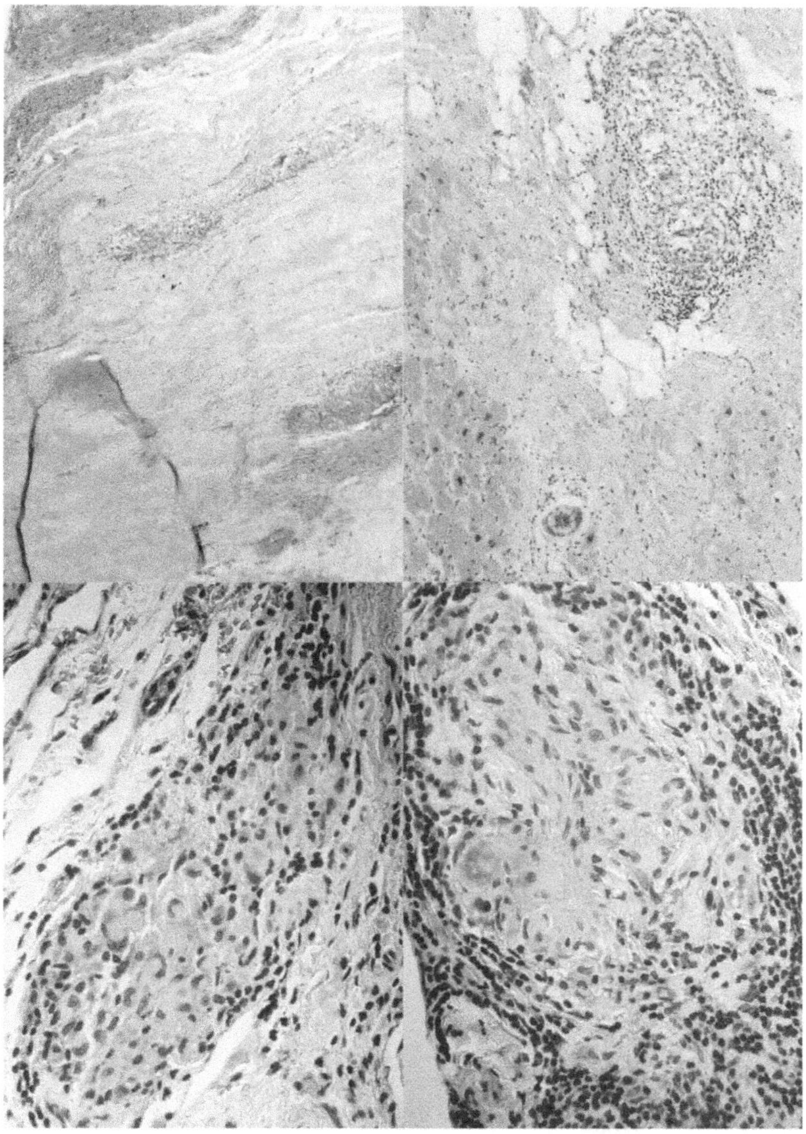

FIGURE 3. Photomicrographs of various portions of the left ventricular wall in the patient described showing typical sarcoid granulomas. *Upper left,* in an area of severe scarring, 3 "hard" sarcoid granulomas are seen. *Upper right,* 1 large and 1 small giant-celled granuloma is seen in an area adjacent to scarring and myocardial fibers. *Lower left and lower right,* 2 granulomas from the myocardial wall showing typical giant cells and epithelioid cells with associated lymphocytes. Hematoxylin eosin stains, X 40 *(upper left)*, X 100 *(upper right)*, and X 400 *(lower left and lower right)*, reduced by 39%.

cephalad portion of the ventricular septum, which is less accessible to biopsy.

Echocardiography may show abnormal wall thickness, left ventricular systolic dysfunction, or pericardial effusion.[10,13] Only 1 study has actually compared echocardiographic findings in patients with cardiac sarcoidosis to those with IDC.[8] In that study of 15 patients with cardiac sarcoidosis, 11 had either thinning (6 patients), thickening (4 patients), or both (1 patient) of the left ventricular wall, whereas only 5 of the 30 patients with IDC had any abnormality in wall thickness. No other differences were noted between the 2 groups. Despite extensive sarcoid involvement in our patient, abnormal wall thickness was not seen on the echocardiogram.

Resting myocardial scintigraphy with thallium-201 may show segmental areas of decreased uptake in up to 30% of patients with sarcoidosis, even those without cardiac symptoms.[14] The unusual feature of these defects is that they tend to disappear after the administration of dipyridamole or on redistribution scanning.[15] Patients with coronary artery disease tend to have fixed perfusion defects or defects seen only after the administration of dipyridamole. Accumulation of gallium-67 is considered an indicator of active inflammation and thus may predict a positive response to steroids.[16] Our patient had repeated nuclear perfusion scans, all of which failed to disclose any resting or exercise-induced defects despite extensive sarcoid involvement of his heart.

Magnetic resonance imaging (MRI) has recently been used to diagnose cardiac sarcoidosis as well as to evaluate the response to corticosteroid treatment.[17–21] Several modalities are available including enhancement with gadolinium.[17] In a patient with biopsy-proved cardiac sarcoidosis, MRI showed multiple discrete, high-signal lesions within the anterolateral and posterior left ventricular wall and septum as well as thickening of the cephalad portion of the septum.[21] MRI has not been systematically compared with other imaging modalities, but case reports have shown the ability of MRI to detect cardiac sarcoidosis when other studies have failed to do so.[18,20] Furthermore, its superior reproducibility makes MRI ideal for follow-up studies to monitor response to treatment.

In summary, this report describes a 53-year-old man who underwent HT for severe heart failure thought to be due to IDC when, in fact, examination of the explanted heart revealed significant sarcoid involvement. Only 2 such cases of HT for undiagnosed cardiac sarcoidosis have been previously reported.

1. Valantine HA, Tazelaar HD, Macoviak J, Mullin AV, Hunt SA, Fowler MB, Billingham ME, Schroeder JS. Cardiac sarcoidosis: response to steroids and transplantation. *J Heart Transplant* 1987;6:244–250.
2. Gokel JM, Reichart B, Struck E. Human cardiac transplantation—evaluation of morphological changes in serial endomyocardial biopsies. *Path Res Pract* 1985;178:354–364.
3. Ankersmit HJ, Wieselthaler GA, Moser B, Taghavi S, Grimm M, Roth G, Gorlitzer M, Tschernich H, Horvat R, Wolner E. Automated implantable cardiac defibrillator and biventricular Thoratec assist

device as bridge to transplantation in a patient with sarcoidosis. *J Thorac Cardiovasc Surg* 2001;121: 1198–1199.

4. Oni AA, Hershberger RE, Norman DJ, Ray J, Hovaguimian H, Cobanoglu AM, Hosenpud JD. Recurrence of sarcoidosis in a cardiac allograft: control with augmented corticosteroids. *J Heart Lung Transplant* 1992;11:367–369.

5. Bernstein M, Konzelmann FW, Sidlick DM. Boeck's sarcoid: report of a case with visceral involvement. *Arch Intern Med* 1929;44:721–734.

6. Gozo EG, Cosnow I, Cohen HC, Okum L. The heart in sarcoidosis. *Chest* 1971;60:379–388.

7. Roberts WC, McAllister HA, Ferrans VJ. Sarcoidosis of the heart. A clinicopathologic study of 35 necropsy patients (group I) and review of 78 previously described necropsy patients (group II). *Am J Med* 1977;63:86–108.

8. Silverman KJ, Hutchins GM, Buckley BH. Cardiac sarcoid: a clinicopathologic study of 84 unselected patients with systemic sarcoidosis. *Circulation* 1978;58:1204–1211.

9. Yazaki Y, Isobe M, Hiramitsu S, Morimoto S, Hiroe M, Omichi C, Nakano T, Saeki M, Izumi T, Sekiguchi M. Comparison of clinical features and prognosis of cardiac sarcoidosis and idiopathic dilated cardiomyopathy. *Am J Cardiol* 1998;82:537–540.

10. Fleming HA. Cardiac sarcoidosis. *Sem Resp Med* 1986;8:65–71.

11. Uemura A, Morimoto S, Hiramitsu S, Kato Y, Ito T, Hishida H. Histologic diagnostic rate of cardiac sarcoidosis: evaluation of endomyocardial biopsies. *Am Heart J* 1999;138:299–302.

12. Ratner SJ, Fenoglio JJ, Ursell PC. Utility of endomyocardial biopsy in the diagnosis of cardiac sarcoidosis. *Chest* 1986;90:528–533.

13. Lewin RF, Mor R, Spitzer S, Arditti A, Hellman C, Agmon J. Echocardiographic evaluation of patients with systemic sarcoidosis. *Am Heart J* 1985; 110:116–122.

14. Kinney EI, Jackson GL, Reeves WC, Zelis R. Thallium scan myocardial defects and echocardiographic abnormalities in patients with sarcoidosis without clinical cardiac dysfunction. An analysis of 44 patients. *Am J Med* 1980;96:497–503.

15. Tellier P, Paycha F, Antony I, Nitenberg A, Valeyre D, Foult J, Battesti J. Reversibility by dipyridamole of thallium-201 myocardial scan defects in patients with sarcoidosis. *Am J Med* 1988;85:189–193.

16. Okayama K, Kurata C, Tawarahara K, Yasushi W, Chida K, Sato A. Diagnosis and prognostic value of myocardial scintigraphy with thallium-201 and gallium-67 in cardiac sarcoidosis. *Chest* 1995;107: 330–334.

17. Shimada T, Shimada K, Sakane T, Ochiai K, Tsukihashi H, Fukui M, Inoue S, Katoh H, Murakami Y, Ishibashi Y, Maruyama R. Diagnosis of cardiac sarcoidosis and evaluation of the effects of steroid therapy by gadolinium-DPTA-enhanced magnetic resonance imaging. *Am J Med* 2001;110: 520–527.

18. Doherty MJ, Kumar SK, Nicholson AA, McGivern DV. Cardiac sarcoidosis: the value of magnetic resonance imaging in diagnosing and assessment of response to treatment. *Resp Med* 1997;92: 697–699.

19. Chandra M, Silverman ME, Oshinski J, Pettigrew R. Diagnosis of cardiac sarcoidosis aided by MRI. *Chest* 1996;110:562–565.

20. Smedema JP, Doubell AF. Cardiac sarcoidosis—the value of magnetic resonance imaging. A case report and brief review of the literature. *Cardiovasc J South Afr* 2000;11:218–222.

21. Riedy K, Fisher M, Belic N, Koenigsberg DI. MR imaging of myocardial sarcoidosis. *AJR* 1988; 151:915–916.

Cardiac Transplantation for Cardiac Sarcoidosis With Initial Diagnosis by Examination of the Left Ventricular Apical "Core" Excised for Insertion of a Left Ventricular Assist Device for Severe Chronic Heart Failure

William Clifford Roberts, MD[a,b,d,*], Travis James Vowels[d], Jong Mi Ko, BA[d], John Edward Capehart, MD[c], and Shelley Anne Hall, MD[a,d]

Three quinquagenarians who underwent insertion of a left ventricular assist device (LVAD) because of severe heart failure and for whom histologic examination of the left ventricular apical "core" (removed to insert the device) showed noncaseating giant cell granulomas typical of sarcoidosis are described. Later, cardiac transplantation showed widespread sarcoid granulomas in the walls of the right and left ventricles and ventricular septum in 2 patients and extensive scarring in the third patient in the absence of coronary narrowing. Previously, 11 patients who underwent cardiac transplantation because of cardiac sarcoidosis had been reported, and in 1 of these patients, diagnosis was also initially made by examination of the left ventricular core excised at the time of insertion of an LVAD. In conclusion, excision of a portion of left ventricular wall to enable insertion of a therapeutic device (LVAD) can also serve as the means of definitive diagnosis of the underlying cardiac condition. © 2009 Elsevier Inc. (Am J Cardiol 2009;103:110–114)

Although it may involve virtually any body organ, sarcoidosis infrequently involved the heart, and when it did, it usually did not cause dysfunction of ≥1 noncardiac organ.[1] Cardiac sarcoidosis was usually not diagnosed until percutaneous cardiac biopsy or at necropsy. Earlier, we reported a patient who underwent cardiac transplantation for severe heart failure and diagnosis of cardiac sarcoidosis was not made until morphologic examination of the recipient heart.[2] We found sarcoid granulomas in the left ventricular apical "core" in 3 patients who had a left ventricular assist device (LVAD) inserted because of severe heart failure. Initial diagnosis of cardiac sarcoidosis by this means is most unusual and prompted this report.

Methods and Results

Pertinent findings in each of the 3 patients are listed in Table 1. All were aged in their 50s and 2 were men. All were mildly overweight (body mass indexes 27.0, 26.5, and 27.0 kg/m^2). Chronic heart failure before cardiac transplantation had been present for 3, 4, and 5 years, respectively. Two patients had transient runs of ventricular tachycardia, including 1 with documented ventricular fibrillation. Two had complete branch bundle block and 1 had complete heart block. All had cardioverter defibrillators implanted and 2 had pacemakers implanted. Coronary angiograms showed the epicardial coronary arteries to be either normal (2 patients) or narrowed <50% in diameter (patient 3; Table 1). All 3 had indirect systemic peak systolic blood pressures ≤100 mm Hg. Two were anemic. Only 1 (patient 2) underwent a percutaneous myocardial biopsy, which was negative for sarcoid. Patient 2 also had biopsy-proven sarcoidosis of the lung 16 years earlier (age 36 years) and had been treated with prednisone (10 mg/day) during all 16 years. Spirometry 3 months before cardiac transplantation showed forced vital capacity to be 2.76 L (59% of predicted), forced expiratory volume in 1 second was 1.78 L (49% of predicted), total lung capacity was 76% of predicted value, and diffusing capacity was 57% of predicted value. Times from insertion of the LVAD to cardiac transplantation were 11, 53, and 522 days. Patients 1 and 3 had never been treated with prednisone or other type of corticosteroid, and diagnosis of sarcoid had not been made before the left ventricular apical core had been examined histologically.

Examination of the surgically excised recipient heart showed 2 to have increased cardiac mass. Both ventricular cavities were dilated in all 3 hearts (Figures 1 to 4). (On pretransplantation echocardiograms in patients 1 and 3, right ventricular cavities were 2.6 and 2.3 cm and left ventricular cavities were 9.4 and 5.7 cm, respectively.) All 3 had extensive scarring in the ventricular walls and 2 had numerous noncaseating granulomas.[3] The patient without noncaseating granulomas (patient 1) in the ventricular walls on examination after cardiac transplantation had extensive scarring and foci of lymphocytes in the areas of scarring.

Cardiac transplantation was performed in patient 1 on January 14, 2005; in patient 2, on July 9, 2005; and in

Departments of [a]Internal Medicine, (Division of Cardiology), [b]Pathology, and [c]Cardiothoracic Surgery and the [d]Baylor Heart and Vascular Institute; and Baylor University Medical Center, Dallas, Texas. Manuscript received August 26, 2008; accepted August 27, 2008.

*Corresponding author: Tel: 214-820-7911; Fax: 214-820-7533.

E-mail address: wc.roberts@baylorhealth.edu (W.C. Roberts).

Table 1
Clinical and cardiac morphologic findings in 3 patients with cardiac sarcoidosis diagnosed for the first time by histologic examination of the left ventricular apical core excised for insertion of left ventricular assist device for severe heart failure

Patient No.	Age at Heart Transplantation	Race	Sex	AF	VT	VF	Heart Block	Hct (%)	Pressures (mm Hg)				CI (L/min/m^2)	EF (%)	ICD	PM	Heart Weight (g)	Location of Sarcoid			Cavity (cm)	
									LV	RV	PA	PAW mean						RV	VS	LV	RV	LV
1	50	W	M	+	+	+	+ (LBBB)	38	127/33	81/19	81/40	51	1.0	10	+	0	604	0*	0*	+*	8.0	7.0
2	52	W	M	+	0	0	+ (RBBB)	26	N/A	N/A	51/23	24	1.6	15	+	+	480	+	+	+	5.2	4.2
3	59	B	F	0	+	0	+ (CHB)	42	N/A	33/11	35/16	24	1.3	25	+	+	371	+	+	+	7.5	5.0

* Sarcoid granulomas present in the left ventricular apical core removed for insertion of the LVAD. The walls of the left ventricle, ventricular septum, and right ventricle in the excised native heart (at transplantation) had extensive scarring, but no granulomas. Focal collections of lymphocytes were present in the scarred ventricular walls.

AF = atrial fibrillation; B = black; CHB = complete heart block; CI = cardiac index; EF = ejection fraction; Hct = hematocrit; ICD = implantable cardioverter-defibrillator; LBBB = left bundle branch block; LV = left ventricle; PA = pulmonary artery; PAW = pulmonary artery wedge; PM = pacemaker; RBBB = right bundle branch block; RV = right ventricle; VF = ventricular fibrillation; VS = ventricular septum; VT = ventricular tachycardia; W = white.

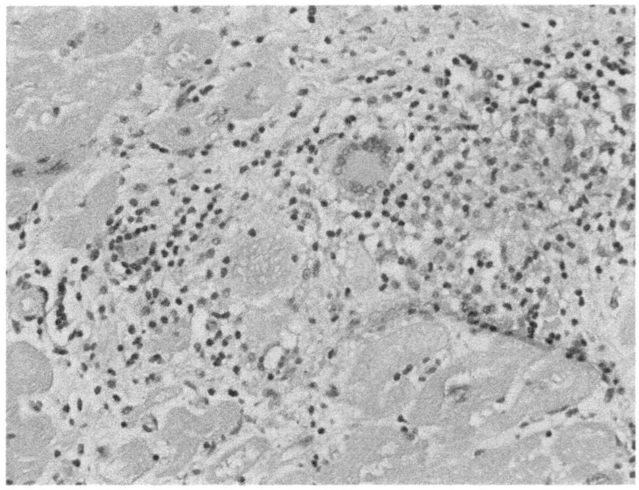

Figure 1. Patient 1. Photomicrograph of sarcoid granuloma in the left ventricular apical core removed 11 days before cardiac transplantation. (Hematoxylin-eosin stain; original magnification ×400.)

patient 3, on July 10, 2006. All 3 patients are alive and active as of August 15, 2008.

The Baylor University Medical Center, Dallas, Texas, Internal Review Board approved the study.

Discussion

The unique feature of the 3 cases briefly described in this report is the initial diagnosis of cardiac sarcoidosis by histologic examination of the left ventricular apical core excised at the time of insertion of a LVAD for severe heart failure of unclear cause. One other patient with a similar diagnostic scenario was reported previously.[4]

We found 11 previously published case reports of patients who underwent cardiac transplantation for severe heart failure (10 patients) or recurring refractory ventricular arrhythmias (1 patient) secondary to cardiac sarcoidosis (Table 2).[2,4–11] Right-sided intracardiac biopsies after cardiac transplantation were reported later in 7 of these 11 patients, and in 2, noncaseating granulomas were found, indicating recurrence of cardiac sarcoidosis, but this time in the donor heart. The positive biopsies were performed 6 and 19 months after transplantation. Biopsies in 5 other patients were negative for sarcoid 6 to 96 months (mean 29) after transplantation. The other 2 patients died 6 days and 42 months after transplantation. Each of the 3 patients described in this report had right-sided biopsies 15, 24, and 14 months performed after cardiac transplantation and none had noncaseating granulomas in the excised cardiac specimens.

Although not performed for cardiac sarcoidosis, Bartram et al[12] reported findings in a 9-year-old boy who developed systemic sarcoidosis (unclear whether the heart was involved) nearly 9 years after orthotopic heart transplantation for Shone syndrome (supravalvular mitral ring, mitral valve stenosis, valvular and supravalvular aortic stenosis, and aortic coarctation).

Zaidi et al[13] reviewed the United Network for Organ Sharing database to assess survival of patients with sar-

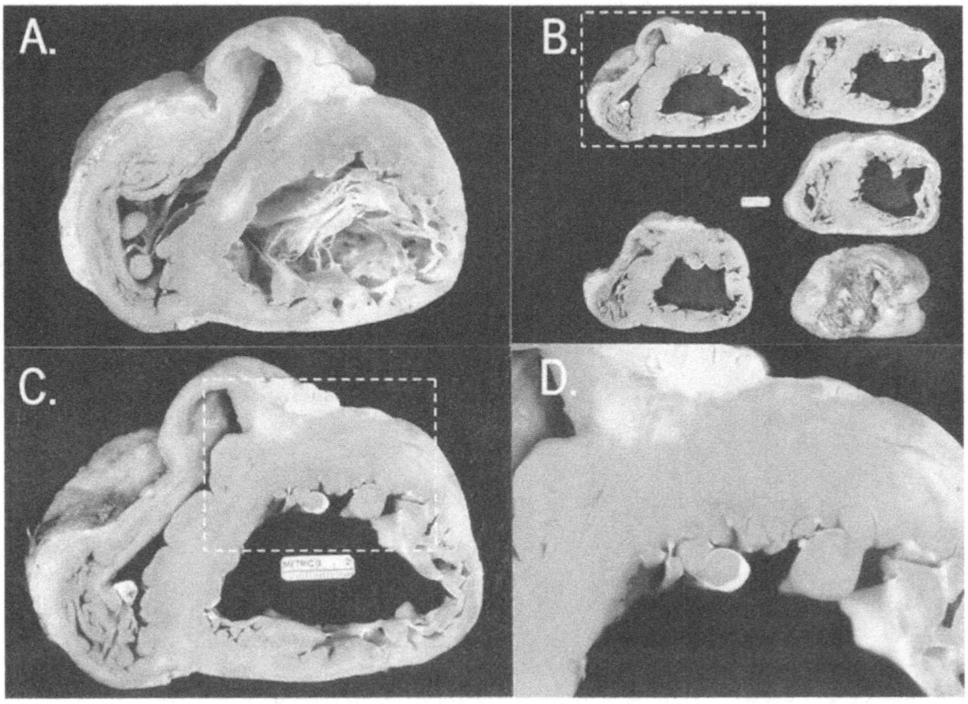

Figure 2. Patient 1. Explanted heart. *(A)* Base shows extensive lateral wall left ventricular scarring and focal ventricular septal scarring by sarcoidosis. Both ventricular cavities are dilated. *(B)* One-centimeter thick slices of the ventricular walls show that scarring extends from base to apex. *(C)* Close-up of 1 ventricular slice shown in *B*. *(D)* Close-up of subepicardial scar in the anterior portion of the ventricular septum shown in *C*.

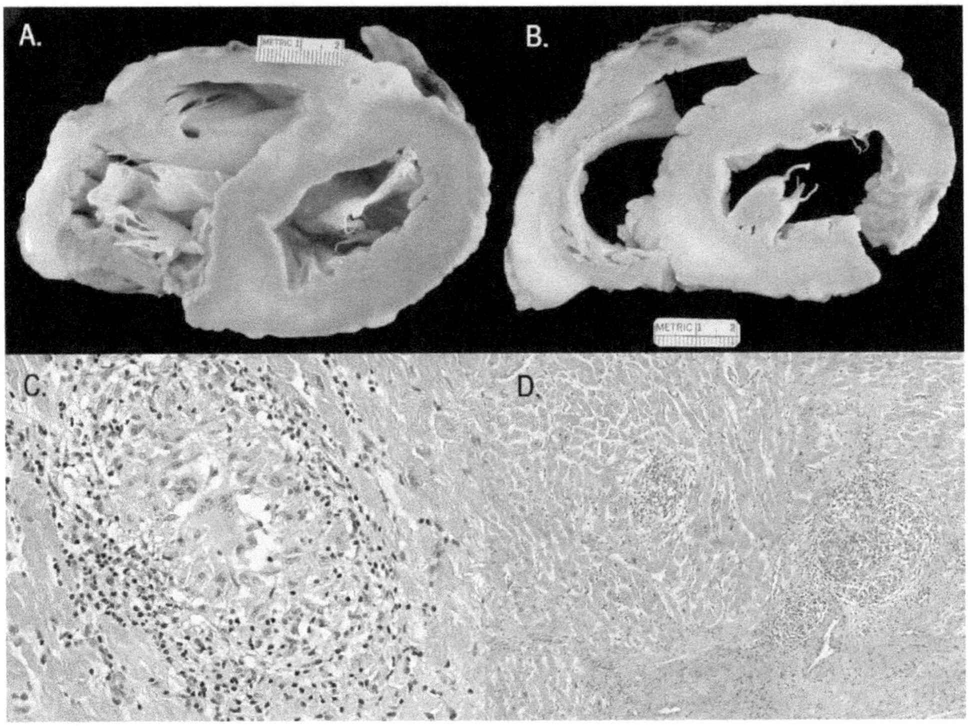

Figure 3. Patient 2. *(A)* Base of heart and *(B)* 1 slice of ventricular walls caudal to the base. Scars are present in the ventricular septum and posterior left ventricular walls. Both cavities are dilated. *(C)* Photomicrograph of a sarcoid granuloma in the left ventricular core removed to insert the LVAD. *(D)* Photomicrograph of portion of explanted heart shows 2 sarcoid granulomas. (Hematoxylin-eosin stain; original magnification *[C]* ×400, *[D]* ×100.)

coidosis treated using heart transplantation. During an 18-year period, 65 patients (40 men, 25 women) with sarcoidosis underwent orthotopic heart transplantation. There were 4 operative deaths and 12 late deaths at a mean follow-up of 40 months. One-year posttransplantation, survival was better for patients with sarcoid undergoing orthotopic transplantation compared with patients undergoing transplantation for nonsarcoid conditions

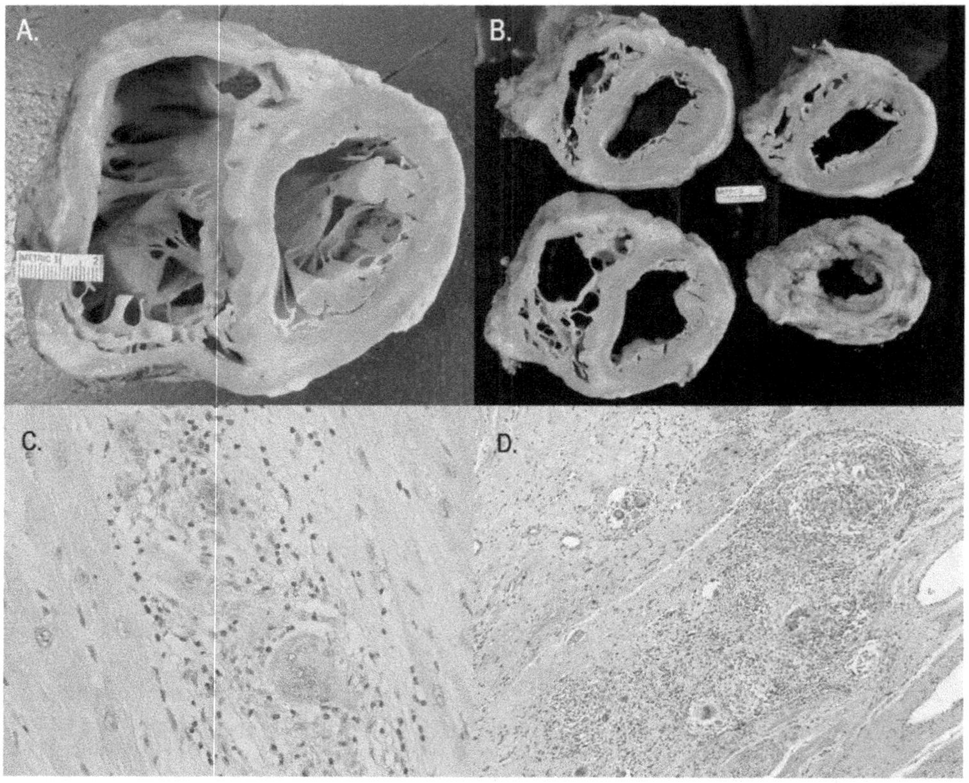

Figure 4. Patient 3. *(A)* Base of heart shows very dilated ventricular cavities and patchy scars in the ventricular septum and left ventricular free wall. *(B)* Slices of ventricular walls caudal to the base again show focal scars. *(C)* Photomicrograph shows sarcoid granuloma in the left ventricular core excised at time of placement of the LVAD. *(D)* Photomicrograph of sarcoid granulomas in the explanted heart. (Hematoxylin-eosin stain; original magnification *[C]* ×400, *[D]* ×100.)

(88% vs 85%; p = 0.03). The investigators concluded that diagnosis of sarcoidosis should not disqualify potential transplantation candidates.

1. Roberts WC, McAllister HA Jr, Ferrans VJ. Sarcoidosis of the heart. A clinicopathologic study of 35 necropsy patients (group I) and review of 78 previously described necropsy patients (group II). *Am J Med* 1977:63:86–108.
2. Donsky AS, Escobar J, Capehart J, Roberts WC. Heart transplantation for undiagnosed cardiac sarcoidosis. *Am J Cardiol* 2002;89:1447–1449.
3. Shirani J, Roberts WC. Subepicardial myocardial lesions. *Am Heart J* 1993;125:1346–1352.
4. Yagar JE, Hernandez AF, Steenbergen C, Persing B, Russell SD, Milano C, Felker GM. Recurrence of cardiac sarcoidosis in a heart transplant recipient. *J Heart Lung Transplant* 2005;24:1988–1990.
5. Gokel JM, Reichart B, Struck E. Human cardiac transplantation—evaluation of morphologic changes in serial endomyocardial biopsies. *Path Res Pract* 1985;79:354–365.
6. Valantine HA, Tazelaar HD, Macoviak J, Mullin AV, Hunt SA, Fowler MB, Billingham ME, Schroeder JS. Cardiac sarcoidosis: response to steroids and transplantation. *J Heart Transplant* 1987;6:244–250.
7. Oni AA, Hershberger RE, Norman DJ, Ray J, Hovaguimian H, Cobanoglu AM, Hosenpud JD. Recurrence of sarcoidosis in a cardiac allograft: control with augmented corticosteroids. *J Heart Lung Transplant* 1992;11:367–369.
8. Ankersmit HJ, Wieselthaler GA, Moser B, Taghavi S, Grimm M, Roth G, Gorlitzer M, Tschernich H, Horvat R, Wolner E. Automated implantable cardiac defibrillator and biventricular thoratec assist device as bridge to transplantation in a patient with sarcoidosis. *J Thorac Cardiovasc Surg* 2001;121:1198–1199.
9. Treaba DO, Benson MD, Assad LW, Dainauskas JR. Sarcoidosis and immunoglobulin lambda II light-chain amyloidosis diagnosed after orthotopic heart transplantation: a case report and review of the literature. *Mod Pathol* 2005;18:451–455.
10. Halushka MK, Yuh DD, Russell SD. Right ventricle-dominant cardiac sarcoidosis with sparing of the left ventricle. *J Heart Lung Transplant* 2006;25:479–482.
11. Greif M, Petrakopoulou P, Weiss M, Reithmann C, Reichart B, Nabauer M, Steinbeck G. Cardiac sarcoidosis concealed by arrhythmogenic right ventricular dysplasia/cardiomyopathy. *Nat Clin Pract Cardiovasc Med* 2008;5:231–236.
12. Bartram U, Thul J, Bauer J, Wössmann W, Schranz D. Systemic sarcoidosis after cardiac transplantation in a 9-year-old child. *J Heart Lung Transplant* 2006;25:1263–1267.
13. Zaidi AR, Zaidi A, Vaitkus PT. Outcome of heart transplantation in patients with sarcoid cardiomyopathy. *J Heart Lung Transplant* 2007;26:714–717.

Table 2
Clinical and morphologic cardiac data in previously reported case reports of patients undergoing cardiac transplantation for cardiac sarcoidosis

Case	Reference	Year Published	Age at HT (yrs)	Race	Sex	Pre-HT Dx of Sarcoid	Reason for HT	Native Heart Weight (g)	Location of Granulomas			Dilated		BBB	CHB	VT	PR >0.20 s	Died (mo after HT)	Recurrence of Cardiac Sarcoid After HT
									RV	VS	LV	RV	LV						
1	Gokel et al[5]	1985	37	N/A	M	+ (Bx)	HF	N/A	–	–	–	–	–	–	–	–	–	+ (8)	–
2	Valantine et al[6]	1987	46	W	M	0	VT	630	+	+	+	0	0	+ [R]	0	+	+	+ (42)	0 (A)
3	Valantine et al[6]	1987	47	B	M	+ (Bx)	HF	420	"Widespread"			0	+	0	0	+	+	0 (16+)	0 (Bx)
4	Valantine et al[6]	1987	51	W	F	0	HF	400	0	+	+	–	–	+ [R]	0	0	+	0 (20+)	0 (Bx)
5	Oni et al[7]	1992	34	N/A	M	+ (Bx)	HF	N/A	–	–	–	+	+	0	0	+	0	0 (13+)	+ (Bx)
6	Ankersmit et al[8]	2001	30	N/A	M	+ (Bx)	HF	N/A	–	–	–	+	+	0	0	+	0	0 (1+)	–
7	Donsky et al[2]	2002	53	W	M	0	HF	510	+	+	+	+	+	+ [L]	0	+	+	0 (105+)	0 (Bx)
8	Yager et al[4]	2005	26	B	M	+ (LVAD)	HF	N/A	–	–	–	–	–	0	0	0	0	0 (24+)	+ (Bx)
9	Treaba et al[9]	2005	53	B	M	0	HF	N/A	+	+	+	–	–	0	+	0	0	+ (0.2)	0 (A)
10	Halushka et al[10]	2006	53	W	M	+ (Bx)	HF	380	+	+	+	+	0	0	0	+	0	0 (6+)	0 (Bx)
11	Greif et al[11]	2008	37	N/A	M	0	HF	N/A	+	+	+	+	0	+ [L]	0	+	0	0 (8+)	0 (Bx)

A = autopsy; B = black; BBB = bundle branch block; Bx = biopsy of myocardium; CHB = complete heart block; Dx = diagnosis; HF = heart failure; HT = heart transplantation; L = left; LV = left ventricle; R = right; RV = right ventricle; VS = ventricular septum; VT = ventricular tachycardia; W = white.

Diagnosing cardiac sarcoidosis clinically without tissue confirmation

Poonam S. Sharma, MD, Jordon G. Lubahn, MD, Alan S. Donsky, MD, Anthony Dong H. Yoon, MD, Melissa M. Carry, MD, Paul A. Grayburn, MD, Prescilla Barrientos Wood, MD, Jong Mi Ko, BA, Elizabeth C. Burton, MD, and William Clifford Roberts, MD

A 52-year-old woman is described in whom cardiac sarcoidosis was diagnosed clinically on the basis of high-grade heart block, recurring ventricular tachyarrhythmias, and acute cardiac decompensation. Confirmation of sarcoidosis was not determined until necropsy. When it causes cardiac dysfunction, sarcoidosis rarely causes dysfunction of another body organ, although small sarcoid granulomas may also be present in noncardiac organs or tissues. In the present patient, neurosarcoidosis accompanied the cardiac sarcoidosis, but it was the latter that produced the life-threatening symptoms and was fatal.

Sarcoidosis is characterized by the presence of noncaseating giant-cell granulomas in more than one body organ. Although these granulomas may be present in virtually any organ, most commonly they occur in the lungs and in adjacent lymph nodes (1), but they are rare in the spinal cord. Symptoms usually appear gradually. Diagnosis often is made by chest radiograph showing hilar adenopathy with or without pulmonary parenchymal lesions before appearance of symptoms. Occasionally, sarcoidosis presents with symptoms related to the heart, and in such circumstances the manifestations usually are acute, consisting of a ventricular arrhythmia or a high grade of heart block or symptoms of heart failure (2). When sarcoidosis causes cardiac dysfunction, infrequently is there dysfunction of another body organ (2). To emphasize the fact that patients with cardiac sarcoidosis severe enough to cause cardiac dysfunction rarely have more than minimal involvement of noncardiac body organs, we describe the following case.

DESCRIPTION OF PATIENT

A 52-year-old nonsmoking, overweight African American female bus driver, who was born in February 1956, had been well until November 2007 when she noted right-sided mid back pain and, in December 2007, impaired vision in the right eye. The right optic disc was swollen and pale. The back pain made it difficult for her to dress herself, it was burning and shooting in nature, and it radiated to her right arm and breast. The impaired vision in the right eye caused blurriness and occasional double vision and was associated with pain with eye movement. Magnetic resonance imaging in January 2008 disclosed multiple small thoracic spine neural foramen tumors and abnormal contrast enhancement in the right retrobulbar fat and along the right optic nerve sheath, and a 15-mm "low-density" lesion in the left lower lobe of the lung was detected by computed tomography. The hilar and mediastinal structures were normal. Treadmill stress echocardiogram disclosed intermittent right bundle branch block throughout exercise and sinus bradycardia at rest, but no ST changes. A four-beat run of atrial tachycardia with aberrant conduction occurred during exercise. No wall-motion abnormalities were seen. Because of the eye problem, she was started on prednisone 80 mg daily and tapered to 10 mg for 7 months. She was off prednisone for the last 5 months of her life. Her vision improved in the right eye from 20/400 to 20/40 as a consequence of treatment.

Repeat chest radiograph in July 2008 disclosed no abnormalities. Echocardiogram disclosed normal-sized ventricular cavities and hyperdynamic left ventricular systolic function. Left ventricular diastolic function, however, was abnormal.

The eye problem cleared and, except for continued periodic right-sided back pain, occasional leg numbness, and some difficulty walking up stairs, she was active and continued working as a bus driver until December 26, 2008, when severe dyspnea appeared. She was found to have complete heart block, and a pacemaker was inserted. The dyspnea, however, persisted and within a week was accompanied by severe substernal chest pain radiating to both arms, dizziness, and worsening dyspnea. She was rehospitalized on January 6, 2009. The erythrocyte sedimentation rate was 76 mm in 1 hour; hematocrit, 31%; troponin, 2.92 ng/mL; and B-type natriuretic peptide, 1183 pg/mL. At cardiac catheterization, the epicardial coronary arteries were normal. The left ventricular ejection fraction was about 55%. Pressures (in mm Hg) were as follows: pulmonary artery, 45/26; pulmonary wedge a wave, 28, v wave, 33, and mean, 26; right atrial a wave, 18, v wave, 23, and mean, 15; left ventricle, 105/14; and aorta, 109/64. A left ventricular angiogram showed a mildly hypokinetic posterobasal wall

From the Department of Internal Medicine (Sharma, Lubahn), Division of Cardiology (Donsky, Yoon, Carry, Grayburn, Roberts), Department of Pathology (Wood, Burton, Roberts), and the Baylor Heart and Vascular Institute (Grayburn, Ko, Roberts), Baylor University Medical Center, Dallas, Texas.

Corresponding author: William C. Roberts, MD, Baylor Heart and Vascular Institute, Baylor University Medical Center, 3500 Gaston Avenue, Dallas, Texas 75246 (e-mail: wc.roberts@BaylorHealth.edu).

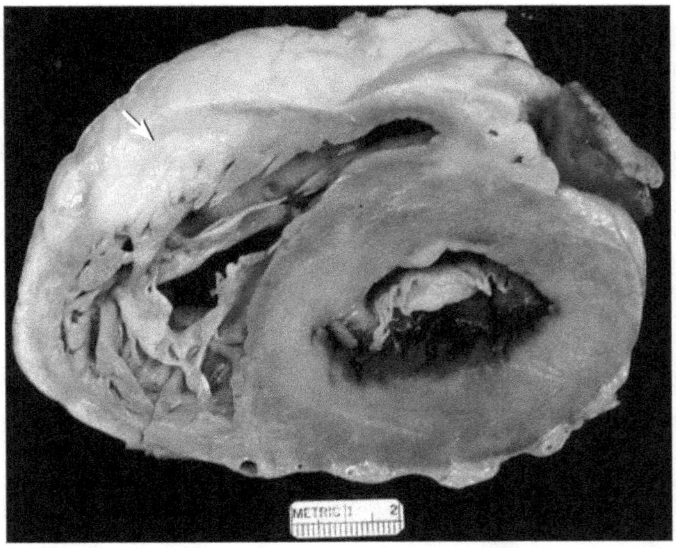

Figure 1. The base of the heart, showing a large sarcoid nodule in the right ventricular free wall anteriorly (arrow).

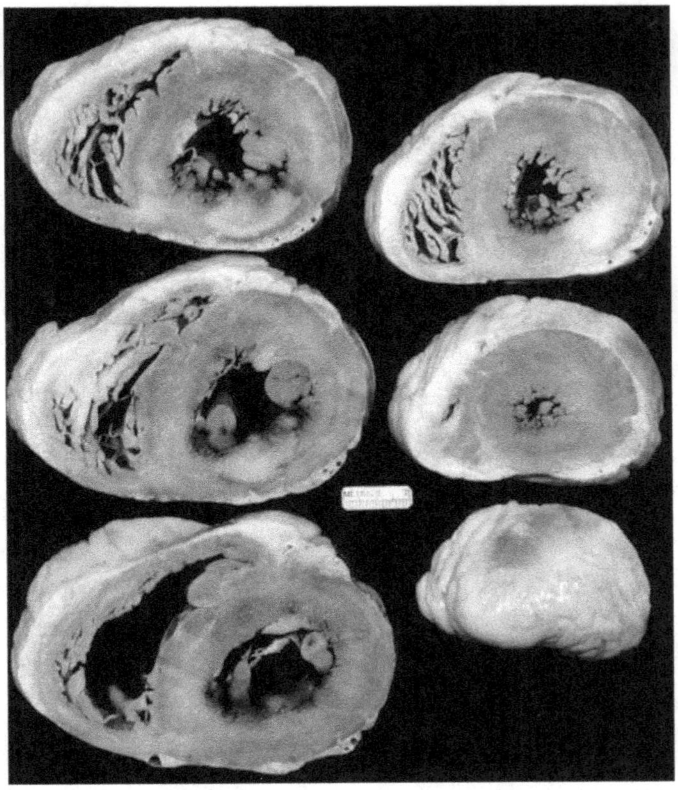

Figure 2. Cross-sections of the ventricular walls and cavities showing multiple sarcoid granulomas. One sarcoid focus involves a portion of the posteromedial papillary muscle of the left ventricle, and this deposit may have played a role in causing the mitral regurgitation.

and 2+/4+ mitral regurgitation. Ventricular tachycardia occurred during the procedure. An echocardiogram on January 16 showed depressed right and left ventricular systolic function (ejection fraction 45%), a restrictive left ventricular diastolic filling pattern, and severe mitral regurgitation. The heart failure progressively worsened, the blood pressure dropped, and ventricular tachycardia refractory to cardioversion occurred followed subsequently by fatal ventricular fibrillation on January 22, 2009.

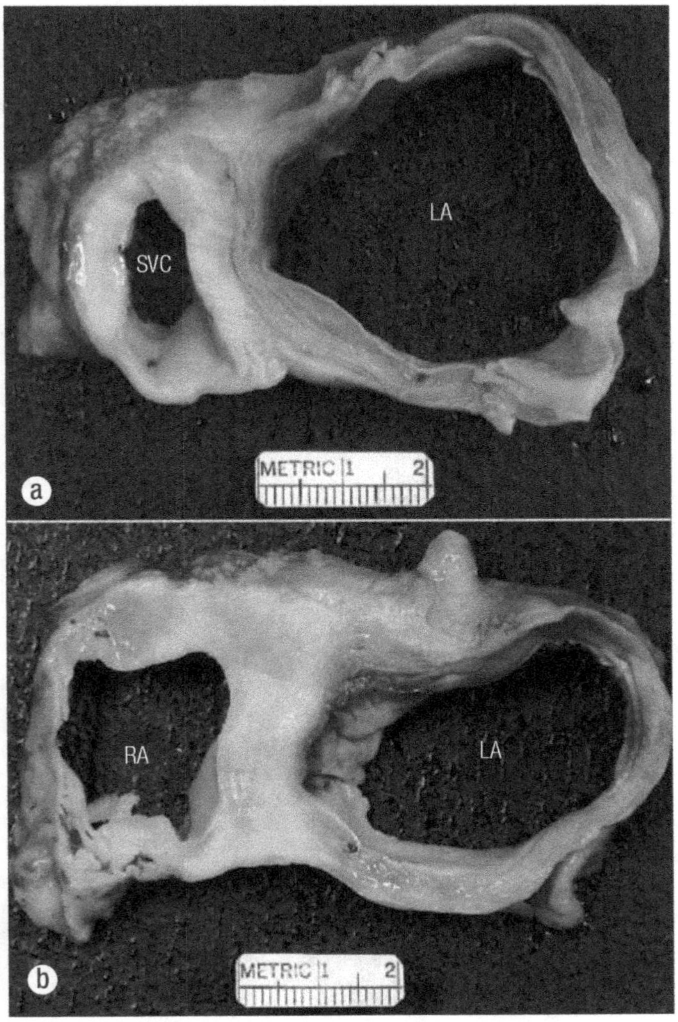

Figure 3. (a) The superior vena cava (SVC) entering the right atrium (RA), with the wall of this large vein replaced by sarcoid granulomas. (b) The more caudal portion of the RA and left atrium (LA), showing sarcoid granuloma in the right atrial wall posteriorly and in the atrial septum.

At necropsy, the heart weighed 485 g. The epicardial coronary arteries were normal. Multiple lesions were present in the right and left ventricular free walls and in the ventricular septum *(Figures 1 and 2)*. Additionally, the wall of the superior vena cava as it entered the right atrium and portions of the right atrial wall and atrial septum were infiltrated by similar lesions, which histologically were noncaseating giant-cell granulomas *(Figure 3)*. Sarcoid granulomas in the right ventricular wall are shown in *Figure 4* and in the left ventricular wall in *Figure 5*. The four cardiac valves were anatomically normal.

The lung parenchyma was normal grossly except for one lesion in the lower lobe of the left lung, and it too was a sarcoid granuloma *(Figures 6 and 7)*. At least two hilar lymph nodes were infiltrated by similar granulomas: one was normal sized, and one about 4 times larger than normal (Figure 7a).

The spinal cord tumors, seen by magnetic resonance, proved to be sarcoid granulomas *(Figure 8)*. Similar granulomas were present in the single kidney (one had been removed earlier for donation to a family member for renal transplantation).

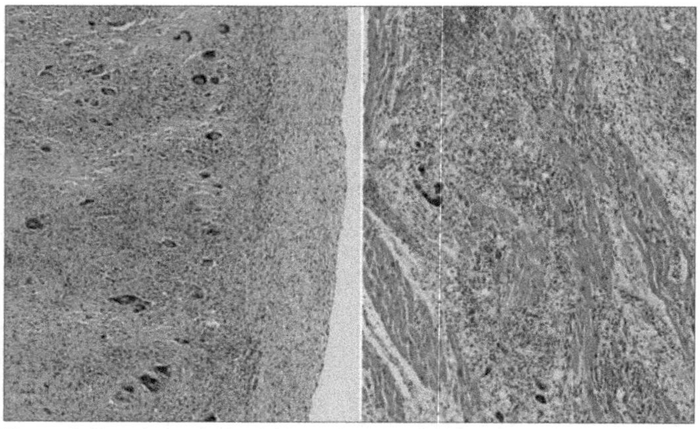

Figure 4. Granulomas in the right ventricular wall. Hematoxylin and eosin stains, each ×100. Stains for fungi and acid-fast organisms were negative.

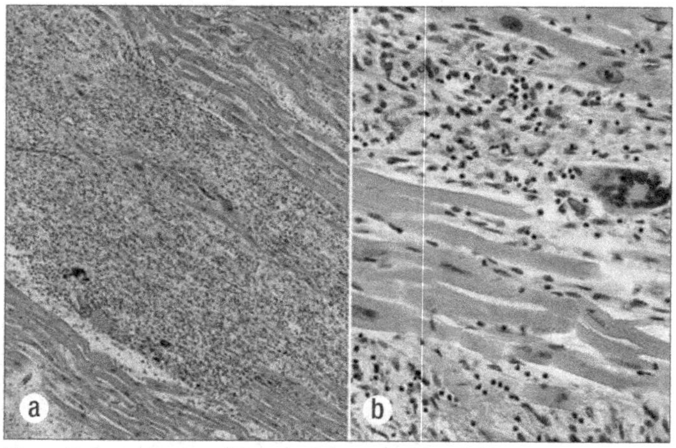

Figure 5. Sarcoid myocarditis in the left ventricular wall. Hematoxylin and eosin stains, **(a)** ×100, **(b)** ×400.

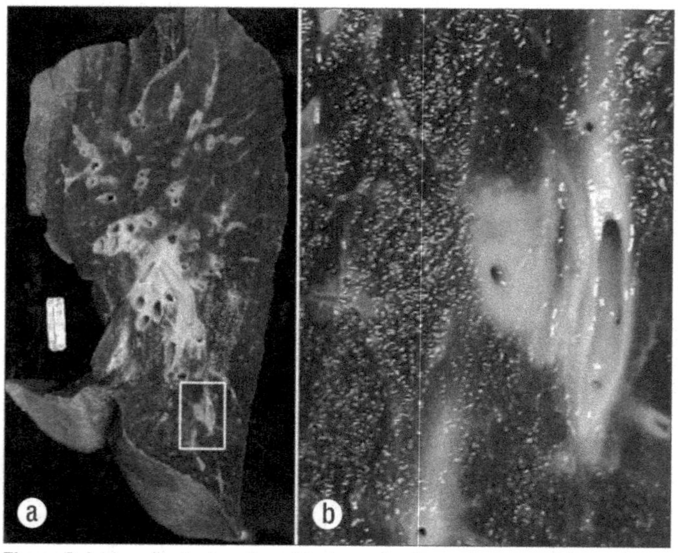

Figure 6. (a) Longitudinal section of the lung showing a single sarcoid granuloma. **(b)** A close-up of the area in the square.

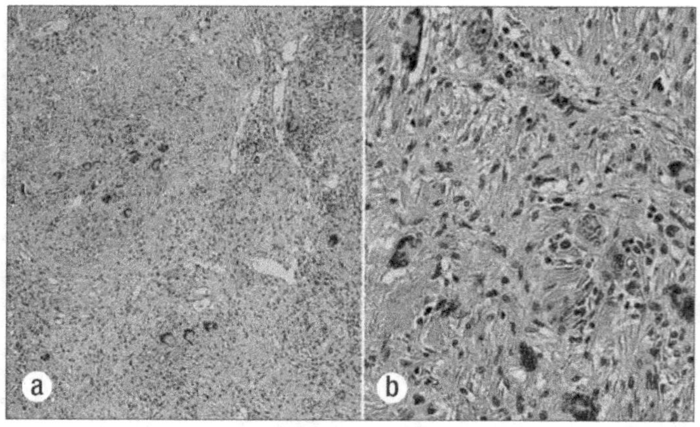

Figure 7. Sarcoid granulomas in the **(a)** hilar lymph node and **(b)** lung. Hematoxylin and eosin stains, ×100 (a), ×400 (b).

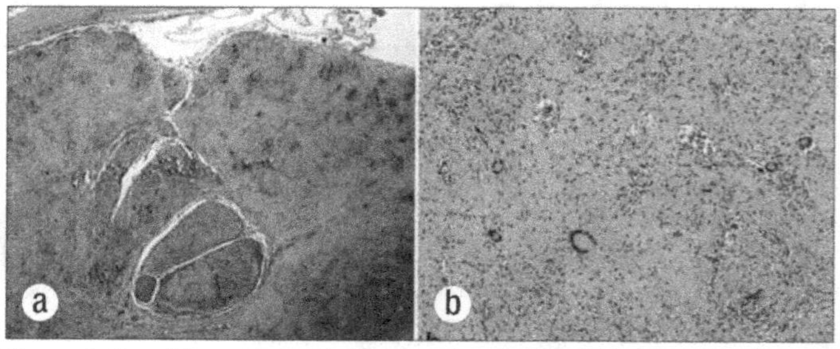

Figure 8. Sarcoid granulomas in the thoracic spinal cord. Hematoxylin and eosin stains, **(a)** ×2, **(b)** ×100.

DISCUSSION

The patient described had classic features of cardiac sarcoidosis, namely a high degree of heart block (third degree), recurring ventricular arrhythmias, and both systolic and diastolic cardiac dysfunction resulting in severe heart failure. Because of this triad of cardiac manifestations, cardiac sarcoidosis was diagnosed clinically. Necropsy confirmed the diagnosis of sarcoidosis, which involved extensively the heart, thoracic spinal cord, and hilar lymph nodes (only one of which was enlarged), and minimally the lung and kidney. The cause of her back pain was sarcoid granulomas within the spinal cord. Although its cause about a year before death was never definitely determined, the visual disturbance prompted the initiation of prednisone therapy, which eliminated the eye problem and obviously is the treatment of choice for sarcoidosis.

A very unusual feature of the present case is the occurrence of sarcoid granulomas in the spinal cord, which led to some nonlimiting symptoms. Others also have reported neurosarcoid involvement in patients with cardiac sarcoidosis (3, 4). Saleh and colleagues (3) reviewed 172 patients with spinal cord sarcoidosis, and 7 (4%) had cardiac involvement. Perry and Vuitch (4), however, found no cases of neurosarcoidosis among 14 autopsied patients with fatal cardiac sarcoidosis.

1. Crystal RG, Roberts WC, Hunninghake GW, Gadek JE, Fulmer JD, Line BR. Pulmonary sarcoidosis: a disease characterized and perpetuated by activated lung T-lymphocytes. *Ann Intern Med* 1981;94(1):73–94.
2. Roberts WC, McAllister HA Jr, Ferrans VJ. Sarcoidosis of the heart. A clinicopathologic study of 35 necropsy patients (group I) and review of 78 previously described necropsy patients (group II). *Am J Med* 1977;63(1):86–108.
3. Saleh S, Saw C, Marzouk K, Sharma O. Sarcoidosis of the spinal cord: literature review and report of eight cases. *J Natl Med Assoc* 2006;98(6):965–976.
4. Perry A, Vuitch F. Causes of death in patients with sarcoidosis. A morphologic study of 38 autopsies with clinicopathologic correlations. *Arch Pathol Lab Med* 1995;119(2):167–172.

Morphologic Features of Cardiac Sarcoidosis in Native Hearts of Patients Having Cardiac Transplantation

William C. Roberts, MD[a,b,c,*], Monica S. Chung, MS[a], Jong Mi Ko, BA[a], John E. Capehart, MD[d], and Shelley A. Hall, MD[c]

Described herein are 10 patients who underwent cardiac transplantation (CT) for severe chronic systolic heart failure resulting from cardiac sarcoidosis. None had the diagnosis of sarcoidosis established before CT except for the 3 patients who earlier had had a portion of left ventricular wall excised for insertion of a left ventricular assist device and non-caseating granulomas were present in the removed myocardium. Although none of the 10 patients had significant narrowing of any of the epicardial coronary arteries, all had focal scarring of the walls of the left and right ventricles and ventricular septum and all had dilated ventricular cavities. The patients with the most ventricular wall scarring tended to have the fewest sarcoid granulomas in the ventricular walls. Two patients had no sarcoid granulomas in the excised heart although one did have typical sarcoid granulomas in the portion of left ventricular wall excised to insert a left ventricular assist device. Patients with cardiac sarcoidosis severe enough to warrant CT had characteristic cardiac ventricular morphologic findings, and no dysfunction of other non-cardiac organs, making clinical diagnosis of cardiac sarcoidosis rather difficult. **(Am J Cardiol 2014;113:706–712)**

Although sarcoidosis of the heart has been recognized for over 70 years, most reports have appeared in the last 30 years. The condition continues to fascinate physicians because of its multiple modes of presentation—ventricular arrhythmias with or without cardiac arrest, various forms of heart block, heart failure, mitral regurgitation, left ventricular aneurysm—and its difficulty in diagnosis.[1–4] Single case reports on the topic continue to appear as well as frequent reviews.[5–12] In the last 2 decades a number of patients with cardiac sarcoidosis have undergone cardiac transplantation (CT) and few of them have had the condition diagnosed before CT or at least before cardiac biopsy (including the histologic examination of a portion of the left ventricular wall excised for insertion of a left ventricular assist device) (Table 1).[13–19] Since 1993, we have studied the hearts of 10 patients who underwent CT for severe chronic heart failure found to be the result of cardiac sarcoidosis. Our purpose was to subjectively quantify the relative density of the cardiac non-caseating granulomas in the myocardium and the extent and characteristics of the resulting scarring in the walls of the cardiac ventricles.

[a]Baylor Heart and Vascular Institute, [b]Department of Pathology, [c]Division of Cardiology, Department of Internal Medicine, and [d]Department of Cardiothoracic Surgery, Baylor University Medical Center, Dallas, Texas. Manuscript received October 15, 2013; revised manuscript received and accepted November 9, 2013.

Monica S. Chung is a second-year medical student at Texas Tech University Health Science Center, Paul L. Foster School of Medicine, El Paso, Texas.

See page 712 for disclosure information.

*Corresponding author: Tel: (214) 820-7911; fax: (214) 820-7533.

E-mail address: wc.roberts@baylorhealth.edu (W.C. Roberts).

Methods

The explanted hearts were sent to the surgical pathology division of the Baylor University Medical Center department of pathology. All hearts were examined and described by WCR and, after "cleaning" and fixation in formalin, weighed, and opened by him. At least 5 sections from the walls of the cardiac ventricles (endocardium through to epicardium) were processed, stained, and examined. From each paraffin block, 2 sections were cut: one was stained by both hematoxylin/eosin and the other by Masson, and each was examined by WCR. The medical records were then examined by MSC, JMK, and WCR.

The quantity of scarring in the left ventricular free wall, ventricular septum, and right ventricular free wall was graded subjectively by WCR on a scale of zero to 4+. Likewise, the density of sarcoid granulomas in the ventricular myocardium was graded zero (none seen) to 4+ (granulomas present in virtually all microscopic fields magnified ×40).

Results

From January 1993 through June 2013, a total of 346 isolated CTs were performed at Baylor University Medical Center. Of them, examination of the explanted hearts disclosed that 10 (3%) had cardiac sarcoidosis. Pertinent clinical and cardiac morphologic findings in them are summarized in Table 2. Their ages at the time of CT ranged from 38 to 55 years (mean 48); 6 were women and 4 were men; 4 of 6 women were black and all 4 men were white. Symptoms of cardiac dysfunction in the 10 patients were present from 1 to 15 years (mean 7). Of the 10 patients, electrocardiograms before CT were available to examine in 9; of the 5 without a pacemaker, total 12-lead QRS voltage varied from 74 to 168 mm (1 mm = 1 millivolt) (mean 132)[20] (Table 2). Body mass index (10 patients) ranged from 19.0 to 32.0 kg/m^2

Table 1
Reported frequency of cardiac sarcoidosis among patients having cardiac transplantation (CT)

First Author (Reference)	Year of Publication	Total CT (Years of CT)	No. (%) With Sarcoidosis	Ages of S Patients (Years)	F/M	W/B	Dx S Before CT	Extra Cardiac Sarcoid	Died	Cardiac Sarcoid Recurrence
Zaidi[13]	2007	38,230 (1987–2005)	65 (0.2%)	4–71 (m 45)	25/40	44/19	—	—	16	—
Miliman[14]	2008	250 (1990–2006)	4 (2%)	25–57	3/1	4/0	1	0	2	0
Luk[15]	2009	296 (1987–2006)	6 (2%)	—	—	—	1	—	—	—
Chang[16]	2012	411 (2003–2011)	5 (1%)	31–40	1/4	—	1	0	0	0
Akashi[17]	2012	825 (1997–2010)	14 (2%)	42–67	7/7	5/7	6	7*	6	2
Totals		40,012	94 (2.3%)	4–67	36/52	53/26	9/1,782	7	24/88 (27%)	2/23 (9%)

B = black; Dx = diagnosis; F = female; M = male; S = sarcoidosis; W = white; — = no information.
* Lungs in all 7.

(mean 25.3). The lowest left ventricular ejection fractions ranged from 10% to 20% (mean 16). Three patients at the time of CT had a left ventricular assist device (Nos 6, 7, and 8, Table 2).

The weights in the hearts in the 4 men ranged from 440 to 605 g (mean 506) and in the 6 women, from 370 to 600 g (mean 476). The maximal internal dimension of the left ventricular cavity ranged from 5.0 to 9.0 cm (mean 6.3); the maximal internal diameter of the right ventricular cavity (right ventricular free wall to ventricular septum at posterior wall at the base) ranged from 2.0 to 9.0 cm (mean 4.5).

Grossly visible scars were present in the left and right ventricular free walls and in the ventricular septum in all 10 patients (Figures 1 to 4) and none of the 10 patients had narrowing of any significant degrees in any of the epicardial coronary arteries. The left ventricular scars were most often transmural but often were also or only subepicardial (outer one-half of the myocardial wall). Scars in the right ventricular free wall were transmural (full thickness scarring). Scars in the ventricular septum also varied in extent: some were transmural and when not were often centrally located in the septum or in the right ventricular half rather than the left ventricular half of the septum. No grossly visible scars or other lesions were observed in the walls of either the right atrium or left atrium, but much of these walls were retained in the recipient to connect to the donor heart. No patient had sarcoid lesions in the cardiac valves, coronary arteries or subepicardial adipose tissue.

The numbers of or density of the sarcoid granulomas in the ventricular walls varied considerably. Some patients had granulomas in virtually every microscopic field magnified ×40 (graded 4+). On the other extreme, 2 patients (#5 and #7, Table 2) had no granulomas in multiple sections of the explanted heart although one of them had typical sarcoid granulomas in the portion of left ventricular free wall excised for insertion of a left ventricular assist device. The patient (#5) in whom granulomas were never observed in the heart had ventricular wall scarring similar to that in the other patients with cardiac granulomas.

An attempt was made to correlate the amount of ventricular wall scarring to the density of giant-cell granulomas in the myocardium. In the 2 patients (#5 and #7, Table 2) without granulomas in the explanted heart each had severe and extensive ventricular wall scarring (grade 4+). Two others (#2 and #10, Table 2) had nearly as extensive ventricular wall scarring (grade 3+) and few (grade 1+) sarcoid granulomas in the heart. Patient #4 (Table 2, Figure 6) had 4+ ventricular wall scarring and 3+ density of sarcoid granulomas in the ventricular walls. The correlation between ventricular wall scarring and the density of cardiac granulomas was less clear in the other 6 patients.

No meaningful correlation was found between the duration of symptoms of heart failure and the extent of left ventricular scarring.

Discussion

All 10 patients included in this study underwent CT for chronic systolic heart failure. In none was the diagnosis of cardiac sarcoidosis made clinically although all 3 patients who underwent insertion of a left ventricular assist device had non-caseating granulomas in the portion of left ventricular wall excised to insert the device. The amount of ventricular wall scarring was considerable in all 10 patients but the number of granulomas in the ventricular myocardium varied considerably in them. Two of the 10 patients had no granulomas in the operatively excised native heart although one of them did have classic sarcoid granulomas in the left ventricular wall removed to insert the left ventricular assist device. One might reasonably question how the other patient without cardiac granulomas was included in the study. The answer is that the quantity of and distribution of the ventricular fibrous tissue in this patient (#5, Table 2) was similar to that in the other 9 patients, none of whom had significant coronary narrowing. The scarring often preferentially involved the subepicardial portions of left ventricular free wall, and also the ventricular septum. Portions of right ventricular free wall were usually involved. We know of no other condition which produces such a distinctive type and distribution of ventricular scarring.

Would diagnosis of cardiac sarcoidosis before CT in these patients with severe systolic heart failure been beneficial to the patient? The answer has not been determined because this diagnosis has been so infrequent before CT.[13–17] Some patients with cardiac sarcoidosis have been benefited by corticosteroid therapy and pre-CT diagnosis would allow a trial of this therapy. Is corticosteroid therapy beneficial after CT for cardiac sarcoidosis? The answer has not been determined. Recurrence of sarcoid in the donor heart has occurred and therefore the answer may be "yes."[21,22]

One feature of cardiac sarcoidosis is clear. Although patients with cardiac sarcoidosis may have non-caseating

Table 2

Pertinent data in the 10 patients having cardiac transplantation (CT) for sarcoidosis

Patient	Age at CT (Years)	Race	Age at Onset of Symptoms (Years)	Duration of Symptoms (Years)	Total 12-lead QRS Voltage (ECG)	ECG Date	BMI (kg/m²)	Pressures (mm Hg)					CI (L/min/m²)	Lowest LVEF (%)	LV AD	Date of CT	HW (g)	Largest Diameter (cm)		Grossly Visible Scar (0–4+)			Density Of LV Sarcoid Granulomas (0–4+)	Figure Number
								PA (s/d)	RV (s/d)	RA (Mean)	LV (s/d)	Aorta (s/d)						LV	RV	LV	VS	RV		
WOMEN																								
1	50	B	38	12	113*	10/05/2008	27.0	—	43/—†	10†	—	—	—	20	0	1/28/2012	440	7.5	4.0	3+	2+	1+	4+	1
2	52	B	48	4	—	—	28.7	59/28	59/15	9	115/34	115/79	1.7	20	0	9/4/2010	440	5.5	2.0	3+	2+	1+	1+	2
3	56	W	55	1	—	—	25.7	—	—	—	109/33	104/79	—	15	0	10/30/2009	445	5.5	3.5	4+	4+	4+	4+	
4	58	W	54	4	74	3/10/2012	26.4	20/11	—	8	—	—	2.2	20	0	3/10/2012	560	5.0	2.5	4+	4+	2+	3+	3,6
5	62	B	49	13	168	2/18/2013	19.0	36/14	62/—†	20†	—	—	2.6	10	0	3/16/2013	600	7.5	6.0	4+	0	2+	0	4
6	59‡	B	55	4	—	—	20.8	44/21	—	—	—	—	1.8	20	+	7/9/2006	370	5.0	7.5	2+	2+	0	4+	6
MEN																								
7	50‡,§	W	47	3	147	1/02/2005	24.7	97/45	92/15	11	—	—	1.7	10	+	1/14/2005	605	7.0	2.5	4+	1+	0	0‖	
8	52‡,§	W	48	4	158*	11/22/2002	21.6	51/23	49/6	6	—	—	1.6	20	+	7/8/2005	440	5.0	3.5	2+	2+	0	4+	
9	54¶	W	41	13	—	—	27.5	32/14	32/12	8	—	—	2.1	10	0	9/5/1999	510	9.0	9.0	1+	1+	1+	4+	
10	63	W	48	15	—	—	32	23/8	24/7	−1	—	—	1.6	15	0	1/6/2013	470	6.0	4.0	3+	1+	4+	1+	5

B = black; BMI = body mass index; CI = cardiac index; ECG = electrocardiogram; HW = heart weight; IC = ischemic cardiomyopathy; LV = left ventricular; LVAD = left ventricular assist device; LVEF = left ventricular ejection fraction; PA = pulmonary artery; RA = right atrial; RV = right ventricular; S = sarcoidosis; VS = ventricular septum; W = white.

* Electrocardiogram recorded 3 or 4 years before CT.

† Values from echocardiogram.

‡ These 3 patients were included in a previous report (*Am J Cardiol* 2009;103:110–114)[19].

§ Diagnosis of cardiac sarcoid made from histologic study of "left ventricular core" excised for insertion of a left ventricular device.

‖ Sarcoid granulomas present in the left ventricular "core" but not in the excised native heart.

¶ Case previously published (*Am J Cardiol* 2002;89:1447–1450)[18].

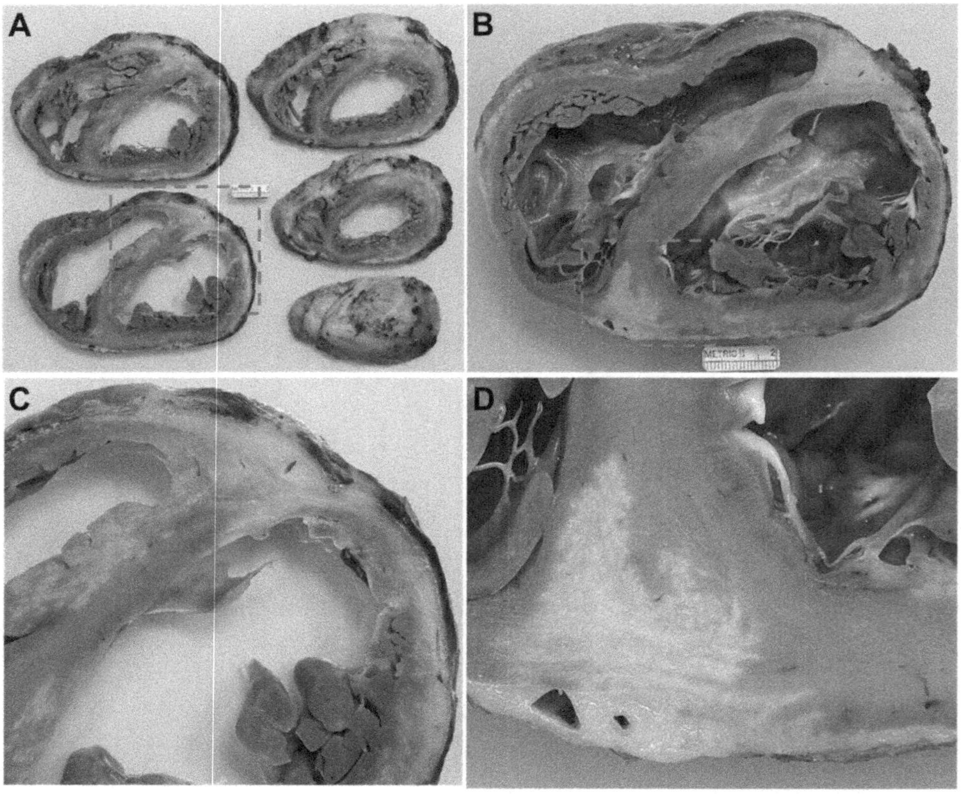

Figure 1. Patient 1, Table 1. Heart in a 50-year-old man who had had symptoms of heart failure for approximately 12 years. *(A)* Sections of the ventricles approximately 1 cm in thickness showing lesions in the right ventricular wall and pectinate muscles, ventricular septum and left ventricular free wall. Some of the scarring, as in the lower left figure of the left ventricular free wall, is subepicardial only. *(B)* Section of the base of the heart exposing the tricuspid and mitral valves, again showing the extensive scarring in the ventricular septum and left ventricular free wall. The anterior descending coronary artery is wide open. *(C)* Close-up view of the anterior wall of left ventricle, right ventricle, and ventricular septum. *(D)* Close-up of the posterior left ventricular free wall showing a large sarcoid granulomatous lesion in the ventricular septum posteriorly.

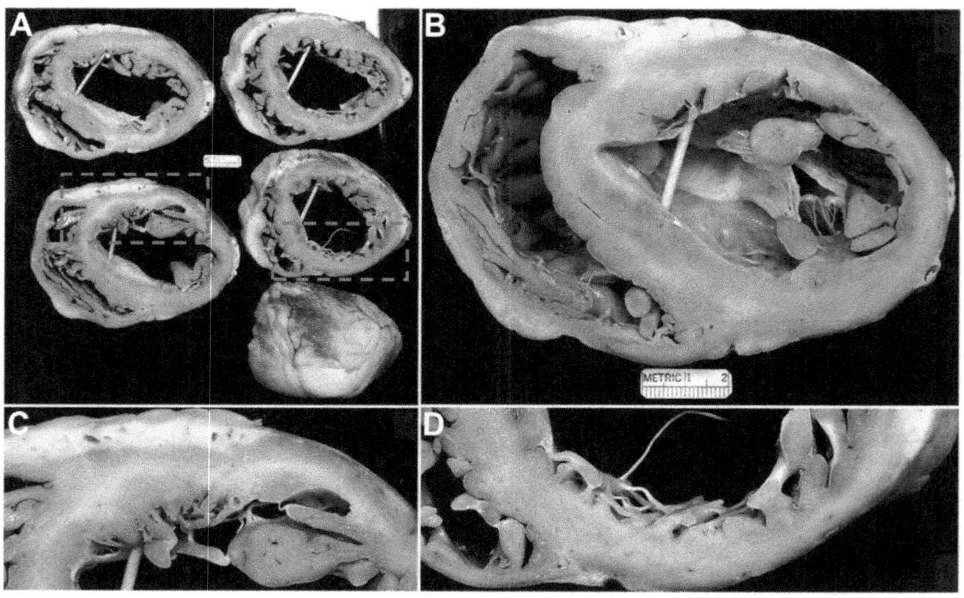

Figure 2. Patient 2, Table 1. *(A)* Views of the various ventricular slices, each about a cm in thickness. Extensive scarring is seen in the left ventricular free wall and ventricular septum anteriorly. *(B)* Close-up of the basal portion showing the mitral valve and the scarring in the ventricular septum and left ventricular free wall. *(C)* Close-up of the anterior left ventricular free wall. The coronary arteries are wide open. *(D)* Close-up view of the posterior wall of left ventricle shown in the brackets in *(A)*. The scarring is mainly subepicardial with relative sparing of the subendocardial portion.

granulomas in other body organs (always in lymph nodes[1]), dysfunction of the involved non-cardiac organ is uncommon. Thus, patients with severe pulmonary sarcoidosis or ocular sarcoid, infrequently have cardiac dysfunction, although an occasional granuloma may be present in myocardium. In other words, patients with sarcoidosis either

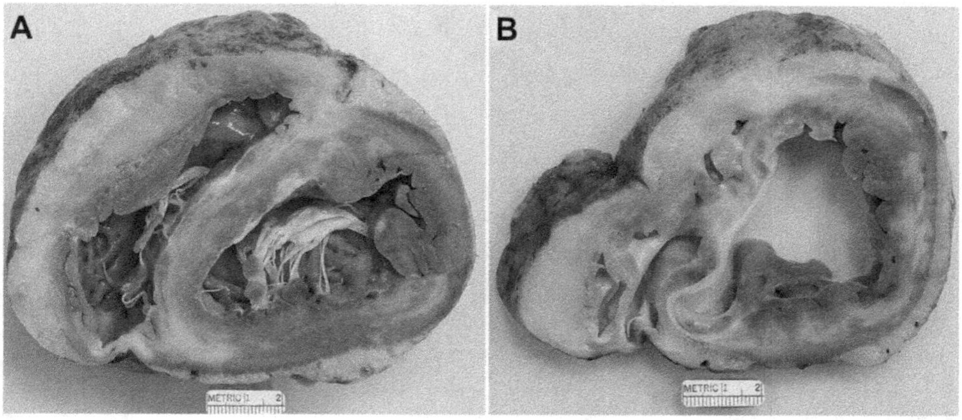

Figure 3. Patient 4, Table 1. *(A)* View of the base of the heart showing extensive scarring in the ventricular septum and also in the left ventricular and right ventricular free walls. Both tricuspid and mitral leaflets are visible. The quantity of subadipose tissue is such that the heart floated in a container of formaldehyde. *(B)* Close-up of a transverse section in the more apical portion, showing an internal aneurysm at the posterior portion of the ventricular septum and left ventricular free wall. The left ventricular free wall scarring is more subepicardial than subendocardial. The scarring in the ventricular septum is transmural.

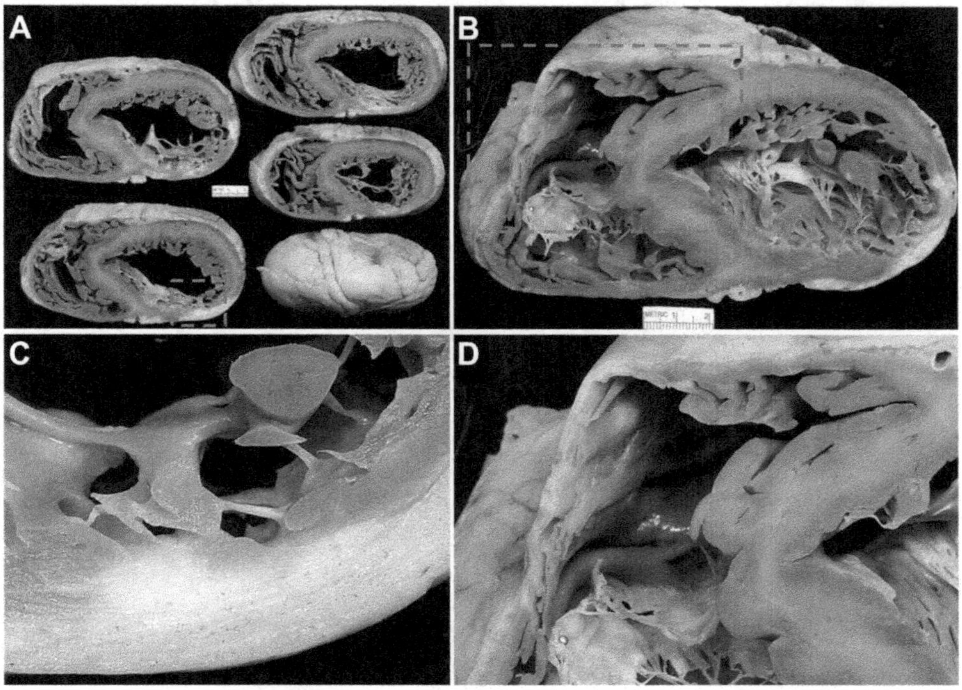

Figure 4. Patient 5, Table 1. *(A)* Transverse sections of the cardiac ventricles showing scarring in the right ventricular anterior wall and left ventricle posterior wall. *(B)* Close-up view of the base showing the tricuspid and mitral valves. The right ventricular free wall is made quite thin by the scarring as is the scarring in the lateral wall of left ventricle. *(C)* Close-up view of the left ventricular free wall showing the scarring to be much greater in the subepicardial region than in the subendocardial region. *(D)* Close-up of the right ventricular free wall showing marked thinning in its anterior lateral portion.

travel the clinical cardiac road or the clinical non-cardiac road, with little to no crossing of the two.

Why is diagnosis of cardiac sarcoidosis so difficult clinically? First, there is nothing specific about the electrocardiogram, echocardiogram, or cardiac catheterization findings. Magnetic resonance imaging and positron emission tomography may be suggestive but biopsy is the only definitive procedure.[23–25] Electrophysiological mapping may be helpful in those patients with ventricular tachycardia.[26] Biopsy of the ventricular septum via the right side of the heart may be negative because the granulomas are focal and can be missed by the biocap. The condition can mimic arrhythmogenic right ventricular dysplasia as demonstrated in our patient #10 (Figure 5) and as reported by others.[27–30]

The positive feature of the present study is the detailed morphologic description and illustrations of the scarring observed in the ventricular walls of these patients with cardiac sarcoidosis. A deficiency is the subjective characterization of the density of sarcoid granulomas and the degree of scarring in the ventricular walls.

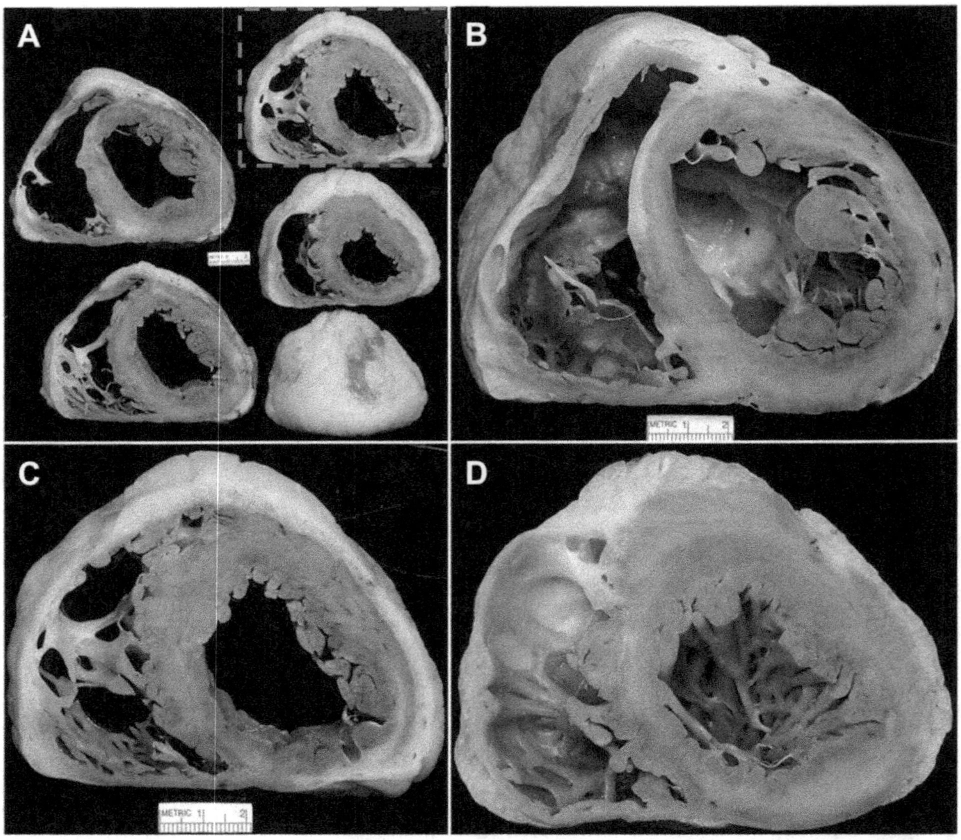

Figure 5. Patient 10, Table 1. *(A)* Close-up views of the various slices of the cardiac ventricles showing extensive scarring in the right ventricular free wall and ventricular septum, and less in the left ventricular free wall. *(B)* Close-up of the cardiac base showing severe scarring of the right ventricular free wall and portions of the ventricular septum and left ventricular free wall. *(C)* Close-up view showing the scarring in the left ventricular free wall to be mainly sub-epicardial. The scarring in the right ventricular free wall and papillary muscle is transmural. *(D)* View showing the severe thinning of the right ventricular free wall anteriorly such that it would assimilate arrhythmogenic right ventricular cardiomyopathy.

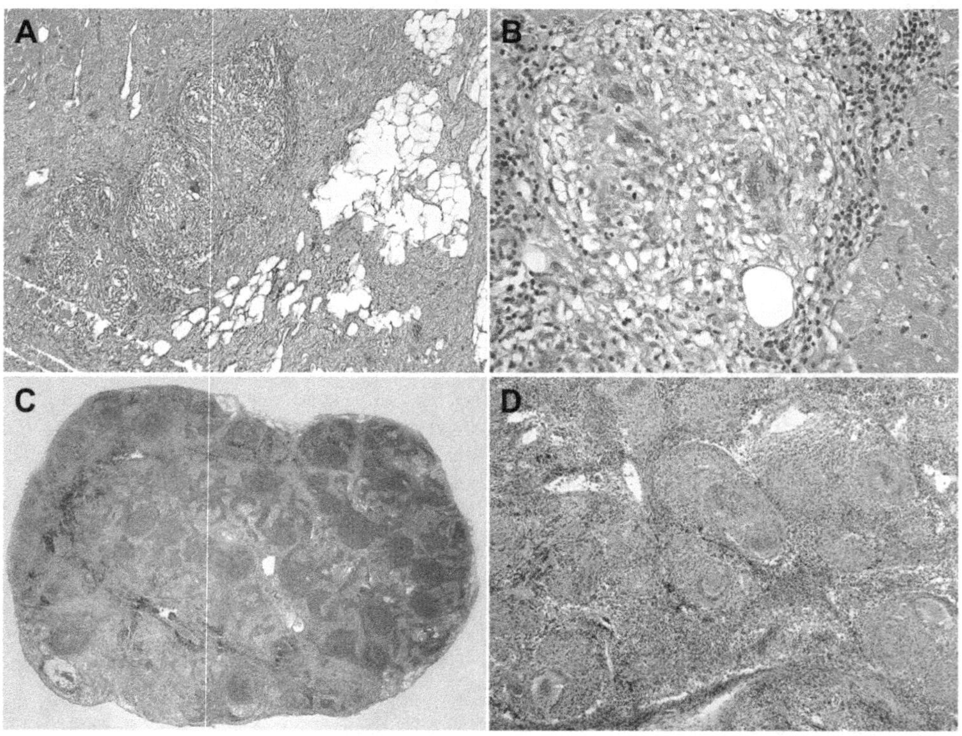

Figure 6. Photomicrographs of cardiac sarcoid granulomas *(A* and *B)* in patient #4 (Table 2) and of lymph node *(C* and *D)* in patient #6 (Table 2). Hematoxylin-eosin stains: *(A)* ×100; *(B)* ×400; *(C)* ×20, and *(D)* ×100. Patient #6 had a mediastinal lymph node excised at the time of CT, the only patient of the 10 to have a lymph node to examine. Giant-cell granulomas typical of sarcoidosis are present in the node.

Disclosures

The authors have no conflicts of interest to disclose.

1. Roberts WC, McAllister HA Jr, Ferrans VJ. Sarcoidosis of the heart: a clinicopathologic study of 35 necropsy patients (group I) and review of 78 previously described necropsy patients (group II). *Am J Med* 1977;63:86–108.
2. Virmani R, Bures JC, Roberts WC. Cardiac sarcoidosis: a major cause of sudden death in young individuals. *Chest* 1980;77:423–428.
3. Sharma PS, Lubahn JG, Donsky AS, Yoon AD, Carry MM, Grayburn PA, Wood PB, Ko JM, Burton EC, Roberts WC. Diagnosing cardiac sarcoidosis clinically without tissue confirmation. *Proc (Bayl Univ Med Cent)* 2009;22:236–238.
4. Tavora F, Cresswell N, Li L, Ripple M, Solomon C, Burke A. Comparison of necropsy findings in patients with sarcoidosis dying suddenly from cardiac sarcoidosis versus dying suddenly from other causes. *Am J Cardiol* 2009;104:571–577.
5. Kim JS, Judson MA, Donnino R, Gold M, Cooper LT Jr, Prystowsky EN, Prystowsky S. Cardiac sarcoidosis. *Am Heart J* 2009;157:9–21.
6. Lagana SM, Parwani AV, Nichols LC. Cardiac sarcoidosis: a pathology-focused review. *Arch Pathol Lab Med* 2010;134:1039–1046.
7. Dubrey SW, Falk RH. Diagnosis and management of cardiac sarcoidosis. *Prog Cardiovasc Dis* 2010;52:336–346.
8. Yeboah J, Lee C, Sharma OP. Cardiac sarcoidosis: a review 2011. *Curr Opin Pulm Med* 2011;17:308–315.
9. Mantini N, Williams B Jr, Stewart J, Rubinsztain L, Kacharava A. Cardiac sarcoid: a clinician's review on how to approach the patient with cardiac sarcoid. *Clin Cardiol* 2012;35:410–415.
10. Saidha S, Sotirchos ES, Eckstein C. Etiology of sarcoidosis: does infection play a role? *Yale J Biol Med* 2012;85:133–141.
11. Hamzeh NY, Wamboldt FS, Weinberger HD. Management of cardiac sarcoidosis in the United States: a Delphi study. *Chest* 2012;141:154–162.
12. Mitropoulos FA, Floudas CS, Kanakis MA, Vaiopoulos GA. Cardiac sarcoidosis. *Thorac Cardiovasc Surg* 2009;57:187–190.
13. Zaidi AR, Zaidi A, Vaitkus PT. Outcome of heart transplantation in patients with sarcoid cardiomyopathy. *J Heart Lung Transplant* 2007;26:714–717.
14. Milman N, Andersen CB, Mortensen SA, Sander K. Cardiac sarcoidosis and heart transplantation: a report of four consecutive patients. *Sarcoidosis Vasc Diffuse Lung Dis* 2008;25:51–59.
15. Luk A, Metawee M, Ahn E, Gustafsson F, Ross H, Butany J. Do clinical diagnoses correlate with pathological diagnoses in cardiac transplant patients? The importance of endomyocardial biopsy. *Can J Cardiol* 2009;25:e48–e54.
16. Chang TI, Chi NH, Chou NK, Tsao CI, Yu HY, Chen YS, Wang SS. Isolated cardiac sarcoidosis in heart transplantation. *Transplant Proc* 2012;44:903–906.
17. Akashi H, Kato TS, Takayama H, Naka Y, Farr M, Mancini D, Schulze PC. Outcome of patients with cardiac sarcoidosis undergoing cardiac transplantation—single-center retrospective analysis. *J Cardiol* 2012;60:407–410.
18. Donsky AS, Escobar J, Capehart J, Roberts WC. Heart transplantation for undiagnosed cardiac sarcoidosis. *Am J Cardiol* 2002;89:1447–1450.
19. Roberts WC, Vowels TJ, Ko JM, Capehart JE, Hall SA. Cardiac transplantation for cardiac sarcoidosis with initial diagnosis by examination of the left ventricular apical "core" excised for insertion of a left ventricular assist device for severe chronic heart failure. *Am J Cardiol* 2009;103:110–114.
20. Roberts WC, Filardo G, Ko JM, Siegel RJ, Dollar AL, Ross EM, Shirani J. Comparison of total 12-lead QRS voltage in a variety of cardiac conditions and its usefulness in predicting increased cardiac mass. *Am J Cardiol* 2013;112:904–909.
21. Yager JE, Hernandez AF, Steenbergen C, Persing B, Russell SD, Milano C, Felker GM. Recurrence of cardiac sarcoidosis in a heart transplant recipient. *J Heart Lung Transplant* 2005;24:1988–1990.
22. Luk A, Lee A, Ahn E, Soor GS, Ross HJ, Butany J. Cardiac sarcoidosis: recurrent disease in a heart transplant patient following pulmonary tuberculosis infection. *Can J Cardiol* 2010;26:e273–e275.
23. Ichinose A, Otani H, Oikawa M, Takase K, Saito H, Shimokawa H, Takahashi S. MRI of cardiac sarcoidosis: basal and subepicardial localization of myocardial lesions and their effect on left ventricular function. *Am J Roentgenol* 2008;191:862–869.
24. Greulich S, Deluigi CC, Gloekler S, Wahl A, Zürn C, Kramer U, Nothnagel D, Bültel H, Schumm J, Grün S, Ong P, Wagner A, Schneider S, Nassenstein K, Gawaz M, Sechtem U, Bruder O, Mahrholdt H. CMR imaging predicts death and other adverse events in suspected cardiac sarcoidosis. *JACC Cardiovasc Imaging* 2013;6:501–511.
25. Khan R, Tweedie EJ, Pflugfelder PW, White JA. Cardiac sarcoid in a heart transplant recipient: detection with cardiac magnetic resonance imaging. *Transplant Proc* 2010;42:1976–1978.
26. Koplan BA, Soejima K, Baughman K, Epstein LM, Stevenson WG. Refractory ventricular tachycardia secondary to cardiac sarcoid: electrophysiologic characteristics, mapping, and ablation. *Heart Rhythm* 2006;3:924–929.
27. Vasaiwala SC, Finn C, Delpriore J, Leya F, Gagermeier J, Akar JG, Santucci P, Dajani K, Bova D, Picken MM, Basso C, Marcus F, Wilber DJ. Prospective study of cardiac sarcoid mimicking arrhythmogenic right ventricular dysplasia. *J Cardiovasc Electrophysiol* 2009;20:473–476.
28. Corrado D, Thiene G. Cardiac sarcoidosis mimicking arrhythmogenic right ventricular cardiomyopathy/dysplasia: the renaissance of endomyocardial biopsy? *J Cardiovasc Electrophysiol* 2009;20:477–479.
29. Chia PL, Subbiah RN, Kuchar D, Walker B. Cardiac sarcoidosis masquerading as arrhythmogenic right ventricular cardiomyopathy. *Heart Lung Circ* 2012;21:42–45.
30. Barbou F, Lahutte M, Gontier E. Cardiac sarcoidosis presenting as an arrhythmogenic right ventricular cardiomyopathy. *Heart* 2012;98:1753–1754.

The Two Extremes of Cardiac Sarcoidosis and the Effect of Prednisone Therapy

Danielle Armstrong, DO[a], Gonzalo V. Gonzalez-Stawinski, MD[b], Jong Mi Ko, BA[c], Shelley A. Hall, MD[d], and William C. Roberts, MD[a,c,d,*]

Described herein are clinical and morphologic findings in 2 patients who underwent heart transplantation because of severe heart failure resulting from cardiac sarcoidosis. Although the explanted hearts in each patient had characteristic gross changes of cardiac sarcoidosis, one patient who had been treated with prednisone, had no residual sarcoid granulomas in the myocardium, whereas the other patient, in whom diagnosis was not made until heart transplantation, had innumerable sarcoid granulomas in her heart. This report suggests that prednisone can eliminate sarcoid granulomas in the heart but that their replacement is by dense fibrous tissue, something also likely the result of the granulomas themselves, creating a situation where the treated (prednisone) and the non-treated sarcoid heart may appear similar by gross examination. **(Am J Cardiol 2015;115:150−153)**

Although it is a systemic disease, sarcoidosis uncommonly affects the heart and when it does the non-cardiac organs are usually minimally affected and they function normally.[1−6] On occasion, cardiac sarcoidosis may lead to such severe heart failure that heart transplantation (HT) is the only reasonable therapy.[3−5] In such situations, diagnosis of cardiac sarcoidosis is usually not made until HT, the usual pre-HT diagnosis being "non-ischemic cardiomyopathy".[5] Recently, 2 patients underwent HT at Baylor University Medical Center (BUMC) in the same month and examination of the explanted heart in one disclosed innumerable myocardial sarcoid granulomas (not diagnosed clinically) and, in the other patient, despite some similar gross findings in the heart, no myocardial granulomas were seen (diagnosed clinically by an earlier biopsy). This report describes findings in these 2 patients to point out the huge spectrum of myocardial changes in patients with cardiac sarcoidosis, and the potential effect of long term prednisone therapy in this condition.

Patients Studied

Pertinent findings in each of the 2 patients are detailed in Table 1. Both patients were in their 50s; both were white; both had severe (4+/4+) heart failure; both had evidence of cardiac dysfunction for approximately 4 years; both had periodic runs of non-sustained ventricular tachycardia; both had some type of heart block (complete in case #1, and right bundle branch block in case #2); neither had dysfunction of a non-cardiac body organ, and neither patient had narrowing of the epicardial coronary arteries. Diagnosis of sarcoidosis before HT was made in patient #1 by biopsy of a mediastinal lymph node 21 months before HT although 2 years earlier a cardiac biopsy had shown "granulomas". Patient #1, who had no granulomas in his explanted heart, was placed on prednisone after the granulomas were seen in the lymph node and he received this drug for 21 months, at very high doses for 10 months before dose-tapering

Table 1
Clinical and morphologic findings in the 2 patients

Variable	Case	
	#1	#2
Gender	Man	Woman
Age (years)		
At heart transplantation	53	57
Onset of symptoms	49	53
Electrophysiology		
Heart block	Complete	RBBB
Ventricular tachycardia	+	+
Pacemaker	+	0
Intracardiac defibrillator	+	+
Systemic hypertension	+	0
Body mass index (Kg/m^2)	31.8	29.9
Hemodynamic data		
Lowest left ventricular EF (%)	20	15
Cardiac index (L/min/m^2)	2.01	1.36
Pressures (mm Hg)		
Blood pressure, indirect (s/d)	100/85	85/40
Right atrial mean	6	2
Right ventricle (s/d)	26/10	48/6
Pulmonary artery (s/d)	26/14	44/11
Pulmonary artery wedge mean	11	14
Prednisone therapy (months)	+ (21)	0
Heart weight (g)	535	380
Cardiac granuloma (0-4+)	0	4+
Left ventricular cavity (cm)	7.5	5.5

EF = ejection fraction; RBBB = right bundle branch block; s/d = peak systole/end diastole.

Departments of [a]Pathology, [b]Cardiothoracic Surgery, and [d]Internal Medicine (Division of Cardiology), Baylor University Medical Center, Dallas, Texas and [c]Baylor Heart and Vascular Institute, Baylor University Medical Center, Dallas, Texas. Manuscript received September 2, 2014; revised manuscript received and accepted October 5, 2014.

Support for this investigation was provided by the Baylor Health Care System Foundation.

See page 153 for disclosure information.

*Corresponding author: Tel: 214-820-7911; fax: 214-820-7533.

E-mail address: wc.roberts@baylorhealth.edu (W.C. Roberts).

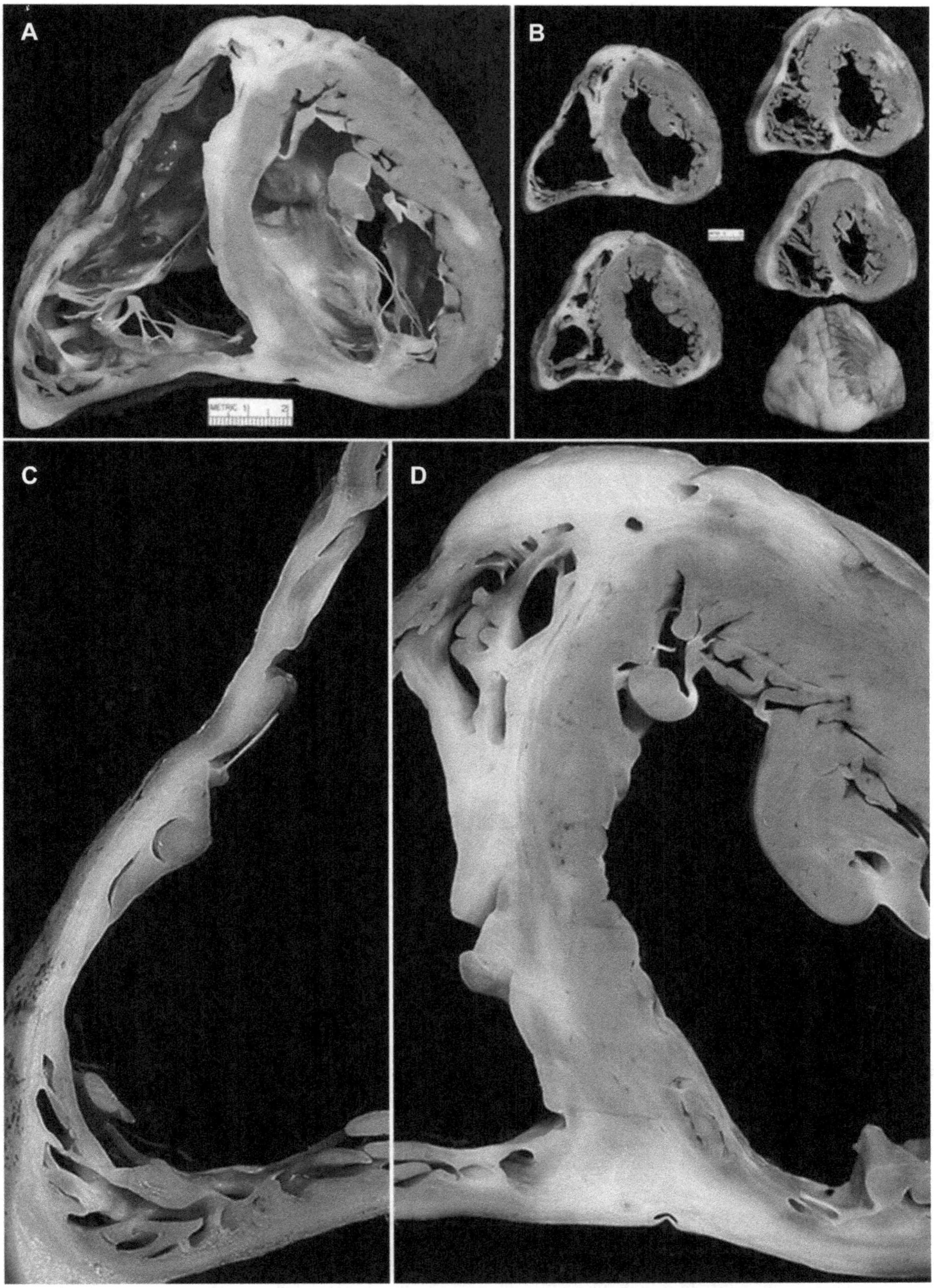

Figure 1. Heart in patient #1. *(A)* View of the base of the heart showing marked dilatation of both right and left ventricular cavities and focal scars in the left and right ventricular free walls and ventricular septum. *(B)* Transverse cuts of the cardiac ventricles caudal to the view shown in *(A)*. *(C)* Close up view of the wall of right ventricle showing extensive scarring and marked thinning of the wall (simulating arrhythmogenic right ventricular dysplasia/cardiomyopathy). *(D)* View of the ventricular septum showing the scarring primarily on the right side of the septum. Because the biotome to biopsy the heart extracts tissue from the right side of the ventricular septum that probably was the reason the biopsy was positive in this patient early in his course.

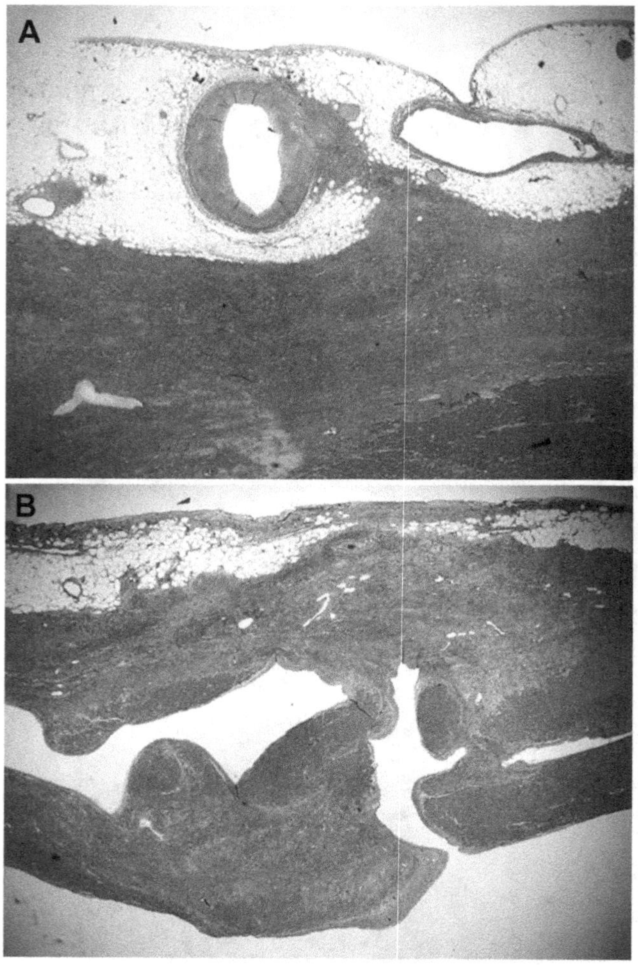

Figure 2. Photomicrographs of portions of the heart in patient #1. *(A)* View of the epicardium, subepicardium, and outer myocardial wall in the anterior portion of left ventricle. The left anterior descending coronary artery and also a coronary vein are shown. The deep blue color represents scar tissue which is located primarily in the subepicardial region rather than the sub-endocardial region. No granulomas were found in the dense fibrous tissue despite examining numerous sections of myocardium. The coronary vessels are surrounded by mainly adipose tissue. *(B)* View of the right ventricular free wall also showing extensive scarring again involving the subepicardial portion more than the subendocardial portion. Trichrome stains, each ×20.

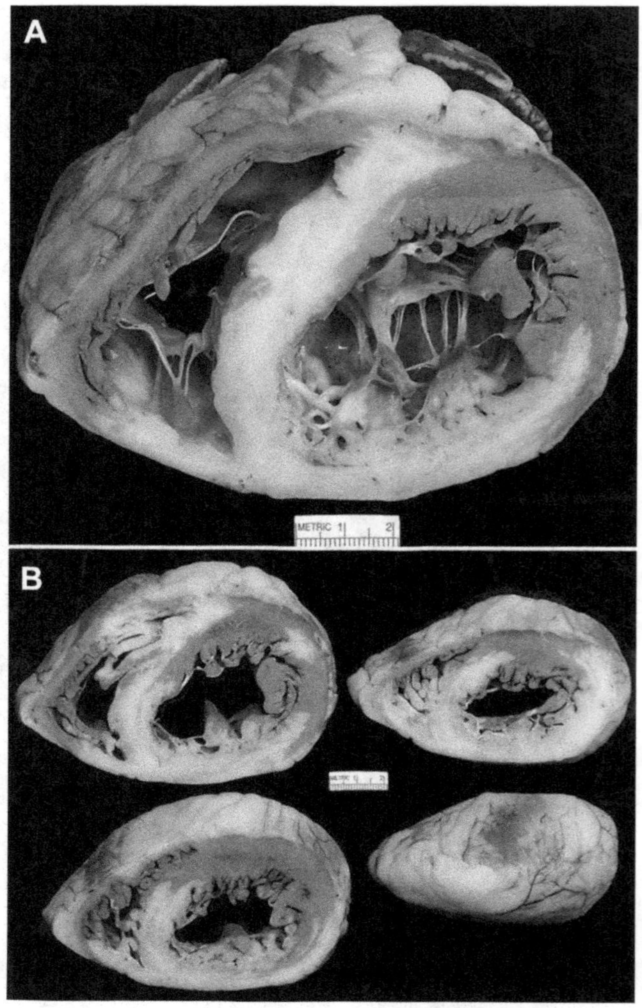

Figure 3. Views of the heart in case #2. *(A)* View of the opened basal portion of the heart showing considerable dilatation of both ventricular cavities and severe scarring of the ventricular septum, posterolateral left ventricular free wall, and posterior wall of right ventricle. Numerous sarcoid granulomas were present in the dense fibrous tissue. *(B)* One-cm thick slices of the ventricles caudal to the upper view. Much of the left ventricular free wall, ventricular septum and right ventricular free wall are replaced by sarcoid granulomas with their surrounding fibrous tissue.

began. Patient #2, whose sarcoidosis was not diagnosed until HT, never received corticosteroid therapy before HT and her explanted heart contained innumerable granulomas typical of sarcoidosis. Photographs of the heart in each patient are shown in Figures 1 to 4.

Discussion

The explanted hearts in each of the 2 hitherto described patients had gross features characteristic of cardiac sarcoidosis: involvement of the walls of both right and left ventricles and the ventricular septum; multiple lesions in each of the cardiac walls; a tendency for the gross lesions to involve the subepicardial half of the left ventricular free wall and the right ventricular half of the ventricular septum, dilation of both ventricular cavities, and absence of narrowing of the epicardial coronary arteries. Yet one patient, who previously by both cardiac and lymph node biopsies showed sarcoidosis, had no granulomas in his explanted heart; the other patient had innumerable sarcoid granulomas in her heart and diagnosis of sarcoidosis was not made until examination of the explanted heart. Patient #1 who had no granulomas in his explanted heart had received prednisone therapy for 21 months, high doses during 10 of those months. The quantity of scar tissue in both patients' hearts suggests that the sarcoid granulomas and their adjacent lymphocytes are strong fibrous-tissue stimulants, and, moreover, that prednisone therapy is a strong eliminator of sarcoid granulomas but the residue of that healing is extensive replacement fibrosis. (Sarcoidosis in the lung is also a strong fibrosis stimulator.[7]) It seems reasonable to believe that the heart in patient #1 earlier had been loaded with sarcoid granulomas as found in patient #2 but that the prednisone treatment likely played a role in eliminating the sarcoid granuloma by replacing them with dense fibrous

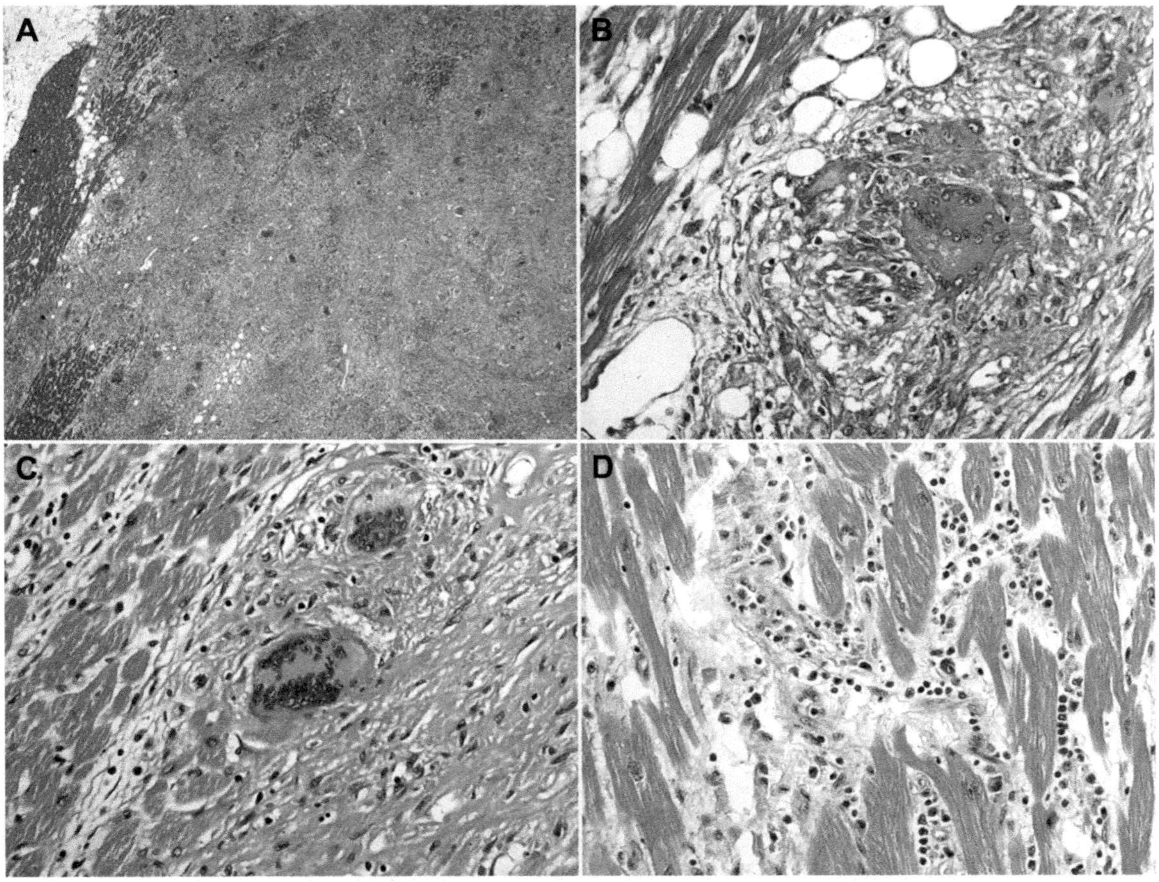

Figure 4. Photomicrographs in patient #2. *(A)* View of a portion of left ventricular free wall showing numerous granulomas surrounded by dense fibrous tissue. *(B)* Close-up view of a single sarcoid granuloma. *(C)* Another view of sarcoid granulomas showing numerous nuclei in each of the giant cells. *(D)* Infiltration between myocardial fibers of lymphocytes typical of sarcoid myocarditis. Trichrome stain, ×40 *(A)*; trichrome stain, ×400 *(B)*; hematoxylin/eosin stain, ×400 *(C)*, and hematoxylin/eosin stain, ×400 *(D)*.

tissue. Such a demonstration to our knowledge has not been provided previous to this report. Earlier we described a patient with typical gross lesions of cardiac sarcoidosis but study of numerous sections of the heart histologically failed to reveal any granulomas.[6] This earlier patient had never received corticosteroid therapy,[6] but earlier histologic examination of a portion of the left ventricular free wall excised to insert a left ventricular assist device did disclose sarcoid granulomas.

Disclosures

The authors have no conflicts of interest to disclose.

1. Roberts WC, McAllister HA Jr, Ferrans VJ. Sarcoidosis of the heart. A clinicopathologic study of 35 necropsy patients (Group I) and review of 78 previously described necropsy patients (Group II). *Am J Med* 1977;63:86–108.
2. Virmani R, Bures JC, Roberts WC. Cardiac sarcoidosis: a major cause of sudden death in young individuals. *Chest* 1980;77:423–428.
3. Donsky AS, Escobar J, Capehart J, Roberts WC. Heart Transplantation for undiagnosed cardiac sarcoidosis. *Am J Cardiol* 2002;89:1447–1450.
4. Roberts WC, Vowels TJ, Ko JM, Capehard JE, Hall SA. Cardiac transplantation for cardiac sarcoidosis with initial diagnosis by examination of the left ventricular apical "core" excised for insertion of a left ventricular assist device for severe chronic heart failure. *Am J Cardiol* 2009;103:110–114.
5. Sharma PS, Lubahn JG, Donsky AS, Yoon AD, Carry MM, Grayburn PA, Wood PB, Ko JM, Burton EC, Roberts WC. Diagnosing cardiac sarcoidosis clinically without tissue confirmation. *Proc (Bayl Univ Med Cent)* 2009;22:236–238.
6. Roberts WC, Chung MS, Ko JM, Capehart JE, Hall SA. Morphologic features of cardiac sarcoidosis in native hearts of patients having cardiac transplantation. *Am J Cardiol* 2014;113:706–712.
7. Crystal RG, Roberts WC, Hunninghake GW, Gadek JE, Fulmer JD, Line BR. Pulmonary sarcoidosis: a disease characterized and perpetuated by activated lung T-lymphocytes. *Ann Intern Med* 1981;94:73–94.

Usefulness of Total 12-Lead QRS Voltage as a Clue to Diagnosis of Patients With Cardiac Sarcoidosis Severe Enough to Warrant Orthotopic Heart Transplant

William C. Roberts, MD; Tiffany M. Becker, BS; Shelley A. Hall, MD

IMPORTANCE Severe heart failure caused by cardiac sarcoidosis is difficult to diagnosis without biopsy.

OBJECTIVE To assess whether total electrocardiographic 12-lead QRS voltage may be a clue to diagnosis.

DESIGN, SETTING, PARTICIPANTS Case-series study with cases collected at Baylor University Medical Center at Dallas, Dallas, Texas, from January 13, 2005, to January 24, 2017. The clinical records of 16 patients with severe heart failure caused by cardiac sarcoidosis were studied. Examination of total 12-lead electrocardiographic QRS voltage (peak of the R wave to the nadir of either the Q or S wave, whichever was deeper) was performed prior to orthotopic heart transplant (OHT). Gross and microscopic pathologic specimens of the native hearts were studied.

MAIN OUTCOMES AND MEASURES The primary outcome was to correlate the total 12-lead QRS voltage measurement with various morphologic features in the native diseased heart.

RESULTS The 16-patient study group consisted of 8 men and 8 women; 12 (75%) were white and 4 (25%) were black. At the time of OHT, patient age ranged from 50 to 67 years (mean, 57 years). Cardiac sarcoidosis was diagnosed by pre-OHT biopsy results in 2 (13%) patients and by examination of the native heart after OHT in 14 (87%) patients. Total nonpaced 12-lead QRS voltage mean was 117 mm (range, 52-155 mm) for 8 patients and total paced 12-lead QRS voltage was 90 mm (range, 67-161 mm) for 12 patients. These low mean values were similar to those of patients with carcinoid heart disease (mean [SD], 105 [40] mm), cardiac amyloidosis (104 [35] mm), and severe cardiac adiposity (120 [31] mm) studied at necropsy or after OHT. In contrast, mean (SD) values were 323 (109) mm in patients with massive cardiomegaly, 257 mm in patients with severe aortic stenosis, 272 (86) mm in patients with severe pure aortic regurgitation, 220 (67) mm in patients with severe pure mitral regurgitation, 197 (64) mm in patients with hypertrophic cardiomyopathy, and 153 (40) mm in patients with idiopathic dilated cardiomyopathy.

CONCLUSIONS AND RELEVANCE Most patients diagnosed with cardiac sarcoidosis causing severe heart failure and warranting OHT had low total 12-lead QRS voltage measurements despite having native hearts of increased weight. This finding may provide a clue to the diagnosis of this disease.

JAMA Cardiol. 2018;3(1):64-68. doi:10.1001/jamacardio.2017.4172
Published online November 15, 2017.

Author Affiliations: Baylor Heart and Vascular Institute, Baylor University Medical Center at Dallas, Dallas, Texas (Roberts, Becker, Hall); Department of Pathology, Baylor University Medical Center, Dallas, Texas (Roberts, Becker, Hall); Department of Internal Medicine, Baylor University Medical Center, Dallas, Texas (Roberts, Becker, Hall).

Corresponding Author: William C. Roberts, MD, Baylor Heart and Vascular Institute, 621 N Hall St, Ste H030, Dallas, TX 75226 (william.roberts1@bswhealth.org).

The first study of the utility of total 12-lead electrocardiographic QRS voltage was published in 1982 and reported findings for patients with aortic valve stenosis.[1] Subsequently, total 12-lead QRS voltage has been reported in a number of other conditions.[2] In each of those studies, the total 12-lead QRS voltage was compared with the weight of the native diseased heart at necropsy or after orthotopic heart transplant (OHT). The present report describes total 12-lead QRS voltage of 16 patients undergoing OHT because of severe heart failure due to cardiac sarcoidosis.

Key Points

Question Is total 12-lead electrocardiographic QRS voltage a diagnostic clue for patients with cardiac sarcoidosis severe enough to warrant orthotopic heart transplant?

Findings In this case-series study, the mean total 12-lead QRS voltage in 16 patients with severe heart failure caused by extensive cardiac sarcoidosis (101 mm) was similar to that determined in patients with cardiac amyloidosis, carcinoid heart disease, and severe cardiac adiposity. In contrast, patients with fatal idiopathic dilated cardiomyopathy had a mean total 12-lead QRS voltage (153 mm).

Meaning The low total 12-lead QRS voltage measurement on electrocardiogram in patients with cardiac sarcoidosis, despite increased weight of the native heart, may be a clue to its correct diagnosis before orthotopic heart transplant.

Methods

From January 13, 2005, through January 24, 2017, 16 patients at Baylor University Medical Center at Dallas (BUMC), Dallas, Texas, had OHT because of cardiac sarcoidosis. The study was approved by the Baylor Research Institute Institutional Review Board, which also waived the need for informed patient consent.

Each patient's native heart was examined by one of us (W.C.R.), and he prepared the final report. Accurate scales were used to weigh the native heart after fixation in formaldehyde for several days. The aorta and pulmonary trunk were excised about 2 cm above the sinotubular junction; all extraneous tissue was removed before weighing. Prior to weighing, the heart was opened and excessive water or formaldehyde was removed from its surfaces by gentle patting with paper towels. Clinical records and all electrocardiograms recorded at BUMC were reviewed and examined. The total 12-lead QRS voltage (defined as the distance in millimeters from the peak of the R wave to the nadir of either the Q or S wave, whichever was deeper) was measured by 2 of us (W.C.R. and T.M.B.). The statistics performed were limited to the calculation of the mean and SD. No statistical package or system was required for these calculations.

Results

The 16-patient study group consisted of 8 men and 8 women; 12 were white and 4 were black. Pertinent morphologic and electrocardiographic findings for the 16 patients are detailed in the **Table** and illustrated in **Figure 1** and **Figure 2**. At the time of OHT, the patient age ranged from 50 to 67 (mean, 57) years. Cardiac sarcoidosis was diagnosed by biopsy in 2 patients (13%) and by examination of the native heart after OHT in 14 patients (87%). The body mass index (calculated as the weight in kilograms divided by height in meters squared) ranged from 18.8 to 32.9 (mean, 27.1). Before OHT, 6 of the 16 patients (37%) had atrial fibrillation; 12 (75%) had bundle branch block (4 with left bundle branch block and 8 with right bundle branch block), and 7 (44%) had complete heart block. The low-density lipoprotein cholesterol levels before OHT ranged from 52 to 147 mg/dL (mean, 93 mg/dL) (to convert to millimoles per liter, multiply by 0.0259). Only patient 12 (Table) had greater than 75% in cross-sectional area narrowing of 1 or more major epicardial coronary arteries (defined as the right, left main, left anterior descending, and left circumflex).

The native heart weighed from 420 to 605 g (mean, 509 g) for the 8 men and from 370 to 600 g (mean, 442 g) for the 8 women. The quantity of cardiac adipose tissue was excessive such that the heart floated in a container of formaldehyde in 7 of the 11 hearts (64%) in which that determination was made. (Cardiac adipose tissue weighs less than myocardium.) Typical sarcoid granulomas were found in the walls of the right and left ventricles and in the ventricular spectrum in all patients. In 1 patient, however, granulomas were seen in the left ventricular wall ("button") removed for insertion of a left ventricular assist device but were not seen in the heart specimen after OHT. The number of granulomas and extent of ventricular wall scarring were subjectively quantified on a scale of 1+ (mild scarring) to 3+ (severe scarring). The distribution of sarcoid lesions is shown in the gross pathologic heart specimens for 3 of the 16 patients (Figure 2).

QRS voltage was measured using a 10-mm standard scale (10 mm = 1 mV) in all 12 leads of an electrocardiogram for all 16 patients. Mean total nonpaced 12-lead QRS voltage was 117 mm (range, 52-155 mm) for 8 patients: 3 men (mean, 137 mm [range, 121-155 mm]) and 5 women (mean, 105 mm [range, 52-144 mm]). Mean total paced 12-lead QRS voltage was 90 mm (range, 67-161 mm) for 12 patients: 6 men (mean, 81 mm [range, 47-103 mm]) and 6 women (mean, 98 mm [range, 67-161 mm]).

Discussion

Described herein are findings from measurement of total 12-lead electrocardiographic QRS voltage and findings from the examination of the native heart in 16 patients who underwent OHT because of severe heart failure due to cardiac sarcoidosis. These low total 12-lead nonpaced (mean, 117 mm) and paced (mean, 90 mm) QRS voltage values are similar to those values previously reported in patients with a variety of other conditions after OHT or necropsy.[2] The mean (SD) total 12-lead QRS voltage for several cardiac diseases is as follows: 105 (40) mm in 19 patients with carcinoid heart disease,[3] 104 (35) mm in 30 patients with cardiac amyloidosis,[4] and 120 (31) mm in 30 patients with severe cardiac adiposity.[5] In contrast, mean (SD) total 12-lead QRS voltage was 323 (109) mm in 17 patients with massive cardiomegaly (weight of native heart, >1000 g),[6] 257 mm in 50 patients with

Table. Pertinent Clinical and Morphological Findings in 16 Patients Who Underwent Heart Transplant for Cardiac Sarcoidosis

Patient No.	Age at HT, y	ECG Paced[a]	QRS Amplitude in Each ECG Lead												Total 12-Lead QRS Voltage, mm	Interval to ECG and HT, mo	BBB (Side)[b]	CHB[b]	LDL-C, mg/dL	SA Pressure, s/d, mm Hg	CI, L/min/m^2	HW, g	Location of Granulomas and Scar			Heart Floated[c]
			I	II	III	aVR	aVL	aVF	V_1	V_2	V_3	V_4	V_5	V_6									RV	VS	LV	
Men																										
1	50	0	7	11	14	5	9	12	6	14	19	7	10	7	121	31	+ (L)	0	119	130/89	1.7	605	0	1+	3+	NA
2	52	0	14	12	8	13	11	7	12	8	8	18	22	22	155	32	+ (R)	0	108	98/58 (I)	1.6	440	1+	2+	1+	NA
3	53	+	7	7	10	4	8	9	5	7	5	6	7	6	81	5	0	+	120	116/66 (I)	1.9	535	3+	3+	3+	NA
4	53	+	4	12	9	6	3	9	7	7	3	7	10	9	86	0.1	+ (R)	+	112	104/70 (I)	1.6	555	3+	3+	3+	+
5	58	+	9	9	6	4	4	6	5	3	8	8	8	7	77	1	+ (L)	0	64	88/55 (I)	1.2	420	3+	3+	3+	0
6	63	+	5	12	8	8	5	10	8	9	14	10	9	5	103	9	+ (L)	+	52	126/78	1.6	470	3+	3+	3+	+
7	63	0	8	6	3	6	6	4	9	10	13	18	22	29	134	34	+ (R)	0	86	120/84 (I)	1.7	540	3+	3+	3+	+
		+	5	8	11	5	6	11	2	4	12	17	11	3	95	2										
8	67	+	4	5	7	2	5	5	2	2	6	5	3	1	47	3	0	+	70	96/59	1.6	510	3+	3+	3+	+
Women																										
9	50	0	6	15	7	9	3	10	7	10	16	16	17	16	132	40	0	+	74	100/60 (I)	–	440	1+	3+	3+	0
		+	2	23	13	6	7	28	4	12	16	20	18	12	161	1										
10	52	+	5	5	5	5	2	8	6	7	7	5	5	7	67	3	+ (L)	0	64	115/79	2.3	440	1+	3+	2+	0
11	56	+	4	7	8	5	6	8	4	8	4	5	7	7	73	0.5	0	0	118	92/64	–	450	1+	3+	3+	+
12	57	0	5	1	6	3	6	4	5	9	5	4	2	2	52	18	+ (R)	0	94	101/58 (I)	1.4	380	3+	3+	3+	NA
13	58	0	8	8	15	3	11	12	5	7	4	4	6	6	89	49	+ (R)	0	147	102/57 (I)	2.2	560	3+	3+	3+	+
		+	3	3	4	2	3	3	3	7	3	3	4	4	69	2										
14	59	0	11	11	17	8	14	13	9	5	9	12	16	19	144	36	+ (R)	+	69	124/92	1.3	370	1+	2+	1+	NA
		+	10	12	19	8	14	15	8	9	10	13	15	14	147	35										
15	61	+	4	4	5	3	6	4	4	10	5	7	7	8	72	0.5	+ (R)	+	60	95/61 (I)	1.2	300	3+	3+	3+	+
16	62	0	10	11	10	7	7	7	10	9	7	9	10	10	107	1	+ (R)	0	129	109/68 (I)	1.5	600	1+	1+	3+	0

Abbreviations: a, augmented; BBB, bundle branch block; CHB, complete heart block; CI, cardiac index; ECG, electrocardiogram; HT, heart transplant; HW, weight of native heart; I, indirect; L, left (or left arm for ECG leads); LDL-C, low-density lipoprotein cholesterol; LV, left ventricle; NA, no information available; R, right (or right arm for ECG leads); RV, right ventricle; SA, systemic artery; s/d, systolic/diastolic; V, voltage; VS, ventricular septum.

SI conversion factor: To convert LDL-C to millimoles per liter, multiply by 0.0259.

[a] + Indicates paced; 0, nonpaced.

[b] + Indicates present; 0, not present.

[c] + Indicates present; 0, not present; and NA, no information available.

Figure 1. 12-Lead Electrocardiograms

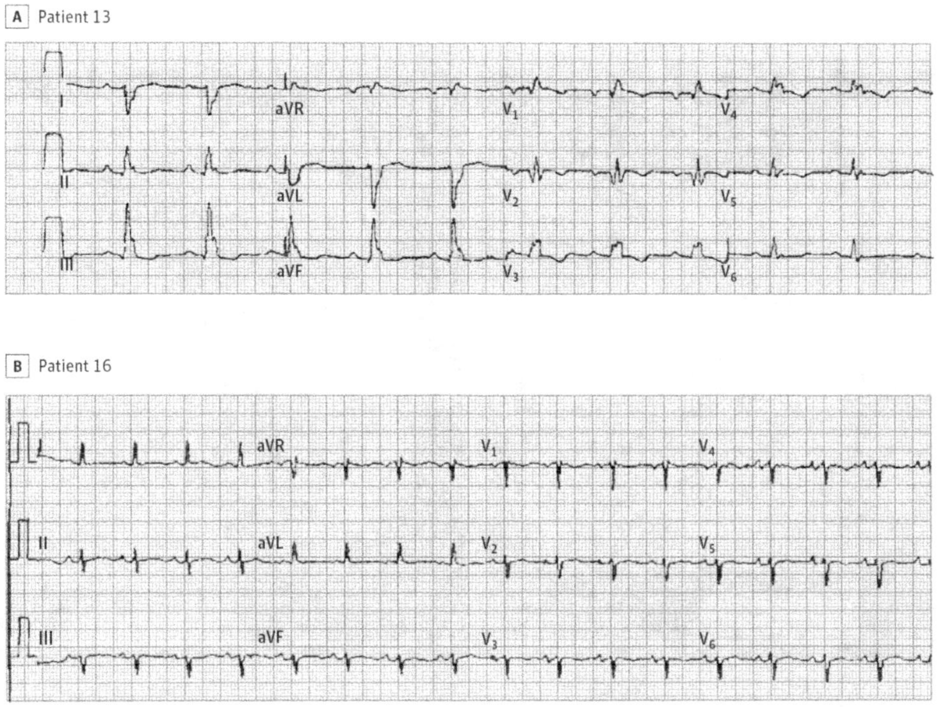

A, Patient 13: total 12-lead QRS voltage is 89 mm; weight of native heart, 560 g. B, Patient 16: total 12-lead QRS voltage is 107 mm; weight of native heart = 600 g. Leads (recording electrodes) are designated as follows: standard (bipolar) leads, I, II, and III; precordial (unipolar) leads, V_1, V_2, V_3, V_4, V_5, and V_6; and augmented limb leads/unipolar extremity leads, aVR, aVL, and aVF (a, augmented; V, voltage; R, right arm; L, left arm; and F, foot).

severe aortic stenosis,[1] 272 (86) mm in 30 patients with severe pure aortic regurgitation,[7] 220 (67) mm in 24 patients with pure mitral regurgitation,[8] 197 (64) mm in 57 patients with hypertrophic cardiomyopathy,[9,10] and 153 (40) mm in 49 patients with idiopathic dilated cardiomyopathy.[11] Thus, most of our patients (15 of 16 [94%]) with severe cardiac sarcoidosis, despite having native hearts of increased weight (>350 g in women and >400 g in men), had low total 12-lead QRS voltages.

Limitations and Strengths

A limitation of the present report is that the time interval between the recording of the electrocardiogram tracing and the OHT procedure was rather long for some patients. It is likely, however, as described previously in patients with idiopathic dilated cardiomyopathy,[12] that the total 12-lead QRS voltage would decrease as the time interval increases between initially developing cardiac sarcoidosis and OHT procedure.[12]

The strong features of the present report are that both the weight of the native heart and the extent of the cardiac sarcoid lesions were known for all 16 patients. To our knowledge, electrocardiographic QRS voltage has not been described previously in patients with cardiac sarcoidosis.[12]

Conclusions

Most patients diagnosed with cardiac sarcoidosis causing severe heart failure and warranting OHT had low total 12-lead QRS voltage measurements despite having native hearts of increased weight. This finding may provide a clue to the diagnosis of this disease.

ARTICLE INFORMATION

Accepted for Publication: September 19, 2017.

Published Online: November 15, 2017. doi:10.1001/jamacardio.2017.4172

Author Contributions: Dr Roberts and Ms Becker had full access to all of the data in the study and take responsibility for the integrity of the data and the accuracy of the data analysis.
Study concept and design: Roberts, Becker.
Acquisition, analysis, or interpretation of data: All authors.
Drafting of the manuscript: Roberts.
Critical revision of the manuscript for important intellectual content: Roberts.
Administrative, technical, or material support: Hall.
Study supervision: Roberts.

Conflict of Interest Disclosures: All authors have completed and submitted the ICMJE Form for Disclosure of Potential Conflicts of Interest and none were reported.

REFERENCES

1. Siegel RJ, Roberts WC. Electrocardiographic observations in severe aortic valve stenosis: correlative necropsy study to clinical, hemodynamic, and ECG variables demonstrating relation of 12-lead QRS amplitude to peak systolic transaortic pressure gradient. *Am Heart J*. 1982;103(2):210-221.

2. Roberts WC, Filardo G, Ko JM, et al. Comparison of total 12-lead QRS voltage in a variety of cardiac conditions and its usefulness in predicting increased cardiac mass. *Am J Cardiol*. 2013;112(6):904-909.

3. Ross EM, Roberts WC. The carcinoid syndrome: comparison of 21 necropsy subjects with carcinoid heart disease to 15 necropsy subjects without carcinoid heart disease. *Am J Med*. 1985;79(3):339-354.

Figure 2. Basal Portions of Native Heart and Photomicrograph of Myocardial Wall in Patients Who Underwent Cardiac Transplant Because of Cardiac Sarcoidosis

A Patient 4

B Patient 15

C Patient 5

D Patient 14

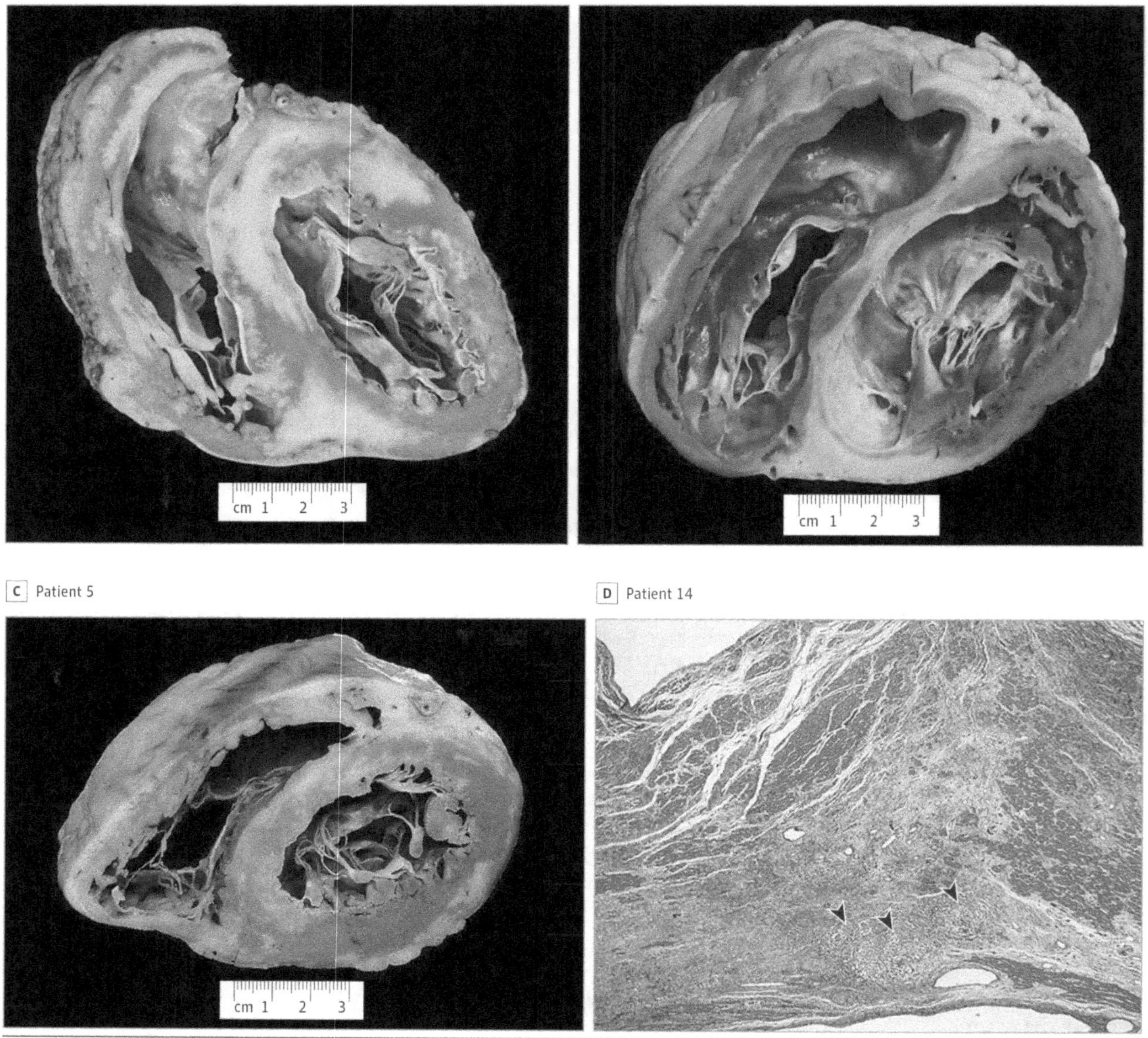

Basal portions of the heart exposing the tricuspid and mitral values. The ventricular septal and left ventricular free wall and a portion of right ventricular free wall contain white lesions; these represent scar tissue within which are sarcoid granulomas. All ventricular cavities are largely dilated. D, Photomicrograph of a portion of the left ventricular free wall of patient 14. The myocardial wall is partially, but extensively replaced by dense fibrous tissue that stains blue and contains several sarcoid granulomas (arrowheads) (trichrome stain, original magnification ×100). Scale bars in A through C are in centimeters.

4. Roberts WC, Waller BF. Cardiac amyloidosis causing cardiac dysfunction: analysis of 54 necropsy patients. *Am J Cardiol*. 1983;52(1):137-146.

5. Shirani J, Roberts WC. Clinical, electrocardiographic and morphologic features of massive fatty deposits ("lipomatous hypertrophy") in the atrial septum. *J Am Coll Cardiol*. 1993;22(1):226-238.

6. Roberts WC, Podolak MJ. The king of hearts: analysis of 23 patients with hearts weighing 1,000 grams or more. *Am J Cardiol*. 1985;55(4):485-494.

7. Roberts WC, Day PJ. Electrocardiographic observations in clinically isolated, pure, chronic, severe aortic regurgitation: analysis of 30 necropsy patients aged 19 to 65 years. *Am J Cardiol*. 1985;55(4):432-438.

8. Glick BN, Roberts WC. Usefulness of total 12-lead QRS voltage in diagnosing left ventricular hypertrophy in clinically isolated, pure, chronic, severe mitral regurgitation. *Am J Cardiol*. 1992;70(11):1088-1092.

9. Dollar AL, Roberts WC. Usefulness of total 12-lead QRS voltage compared with other criteria for determining left ventricular hypertrophy in hypertrophic cardiomyopathy: analysis of 57 patients studied at necropsy. *Am J Med*. 1989;87(4):377-381.

10. Shirani J, Maron BJ, Cannon RO III, Shahin S, Roberts WC. Clinicopathologic features of hypertrophic cardiomyopathy managed by cardiac transplantation. *Am J Cardiol*. 1993;72(5):434-440.

11. Roberts WC, Siegel RJ, McManus BM. Idiopathic dilated cardiomyopathy: analysis of 152 necropsy patients. *Am J Cardiol*. 1987;60(16):1340-1355.

12. Wilensky RL, Yudelman P, Cohen AI, et al. Serial electrocardiographic changes in idiopathic dilated cardiomyopathy confirmed at necropsy. *Am J Cardiol*. 1988;62(4):276-283.

Comparison of Clinical and Morphologic Findings in Patients With Cardiac Sarcoidosis Severe Enough to Warrant Heart Transplantation in Those With -vs- Those Without Non-Caseating Granulomas in the Explanted Heart (Burnt-Out Sarcoid)

Samreen Fathima, MBBS[a,b], and William C. Roberts, MD[a,b,*]

Can cardiac sarcoidosis with heart failure severe enough to warrant orthotopic heart transplantation (OHT) be present without non-caseating granulomas in the explanted heart? The objective is to compare clinical and morphological features in patients with cardiac sarcoidosis severe enough to warrant OHT with -vs-without non-caseating granulomas in the explanted heart. The study was conducted at Baylor University Medical Center in Dallas, Texas. From a total of 671 explanted hearts examined from 1993 to 2018, twenty-five (4%) had gross morphologic features characteristic of cardiac sarcoidosis. At the time of OHT, the patients ranged in age from 50 to 69 years [mean 57]. Cardiac sarcoidosis was diagnosed before OHT in 3 (12%) patients, by percutaneous biopsy of the heart in 2 patients and by histologic examination of the "left ventricular core" in 1 patient who had a left ventricular assist device inserted, and, by examination of the native heart after OHT in the remaining 22 (88%) patients. Of the 25 patients, 16 (64%) had typical sarcoid non-caseating granulomas in the explanted heart, and 9 (36%) had no granulomas in the explanted heart. Comparison of certain clinical and morphologic features in the group with -vs- the group without cardiac granulomas showed no significant differences. In conclusion, of patients with cardiac sarcoidosis severe enough to warrant OHT, some have typical non-caseating granulomas in the explanted heart and some do not. The clinical and gross morphologic features of those with and those without cardiac granulomas are similar. **(Am J Cardiol 2019;124:599−603)**

Sarcoidosis has usually been defined by the presence of non-caseating granulomas containing multinucleated giant cells, epithelioid cells and lymphocytes in one or more body organs. When sarcoidosis attacks an organ, scar tissue develops in the areas of the granulomas and eventually it appears that the scar tissue can obliterate all evidence of previous inflammation, including the giant cells. This scenario appears to occur in cardiac sarcoidosis. Herein, we describe certain clinical and cardiac morphologic findings in 25 patients who had orthotopic heart transplant (OHT) for what proved to be cardiac sarcoidosis. We compared clinical and morphologic features of the cases with to those without non-caseating granulomas in the explanted hearts.

Methods

Since March 1993 one of us (WCR) has examined all specimens excised by cardiac surgeons at Baylor University Medical Center (BUMC) and submitted the report on each. From March 1993 through December 2018, we examined 671 native hearts excised at the time of OHT at BUMC. All hearts were opened and sections made by WCR. The weights of the hearts were all done by the same investigator after opening the chambers, removing any excess tissue (parietal pericardium for example), and incising the aorta and pulmonary trunk about 2 cm cephalad to the sino-tubular junction. The hearts were weighed within one week after their fixation in formaldehyde. Photographs were prepared on virtually all the explanted hearts, all of which have been retained. Of these 671 native hearts examined since 1993, twenty-five (4%) had gross morphologic features characteristic of cardiac sarcoidosis. Histologic sections were prepared in each heart, and stained by both hematoxylin/eosin and trichrome. At least 5 sections of myocardium were prepared in each case: 4 from the ventricles and 1 from the atria. All sections were examined by WCR. Photomicrographs were prepared from many of the cases. After examination of the heart and before submitting the final pathology report, the medical records in each case were examined.

Results

Of the 25 cases, 16 (64%) had typical sarcoid non-caseating granulomas in the explanted heart, and 9 (36%) had no granulomas in the explanted heart. Comparison of

[a]Division of Cardiology, Departments of Internal Medicine, Baylor Scott & White Heart and Vascular Institute, Baylor University Medical Center, Baylor Scott & White Health, Dallas, Texas; and [b]Department of Pathology, Baylor Scott & White Heart and Vascular Institute, Baylor University Medical Center, Baylor Scott & White Health, Dallas, Texas. Manuscript received April 19, 2019; revised manuscript received and accepted May 7, 2019.

*Corresponding author: Tel: (214) 820-7911.

E-mail address: William.Roberts1@bswhealth.org (W.C. Roberts).

certain clinical and gross morphologic features in the group with -vs- the group without cardiac granulomas showed no significant differences (Table 1). Pertinent data in each of the 25 patients is tabulated in Table 2. Three patients (cases #2, #11 and #18 Table 2) had left ventricular assist devices inserted before OHT and all 3 had granulomas in the excised "left ventricular core", including one (case #18, Table 2) who did not have granulomas in the explanted heart. Of the 9 patients without granulomas in the explanted heart, 3 previously had morphologic proof of cardiac sarcoidosis (2 by percutaneous biopsies of the heart [cases #19 and #22, Table 2] and one by examination of the portion of left ventricular free wall excised to insert a left ventricular assist device [case #18, Table 2].) Each of these 3 patients in whom cardiac sarcoidosis was proven by tissue examination before OHT were treated with corticosteroid therapy (cases #18, #19, and #22, Table 2). Additionally, two of the remaining 22 patients in whom the diagnosis of cardiac sarcoidosis was not proven before OHT also were treated with corticosteroid drugs because of biopsy proved pulmonary sarcoidosis (Cases #2 and #24, Table 2). Two patients (case #4 and #7, Table 2) had significant coronary narrowing, one (case #4, Table 2) of whom had coronary artery bypass grafting. Electrocardiographic features before OHT in each of the 25 patients are tabulated in table 3.

Table 1
Comparison in patients with clinical and morphologic findings of cardiac sarcoidosis severe enough to warrant heart transplantation in those with -vs- those without non-caseating granulomas in the explanted heart

Variable	Total (n = 25)	Cardiac granulomas		p Value
		No (n = 9)	Yes (n = 16)	
Age (years)	57 ± 6	56 ± 9	57 ± 5	0.81
Men	13 (52%)	6 (67%)	7 (44%)	0.41
Women	12 (48%)	3 (33%)	9 (56%)	
White	19 (76%)	6 (67%)	13 (81%)	0.63
Black	6 (24%)	3 (33%)	3 (19%)	
Duration (months), symptoms	72 ± 53	76 ± 65	70 ± 48	0.79
Atrial arrhythmias	7 (28%)	4 (44%)	3 (20%)	0.36
Ventricular arrhythmias	8 (32%)	1 (11%)	7 (47%)	0.18
Bundle branch block				0.28
Left	4 (16%)	1 (11%)	3 (19%)	
Right	10 (40%)	3 (33%)	7 (44%)	
Indeterminate	3 (12%)	0	3 (19%)	
Total 12-lead QRS Voltage (mm)	88 ± 36	99 ± 20	82 ± 41	0.30
Total cholesterol (mg/dl)	150 ± 42	160 ± 47	145 ± 40	0.44
LDL cholesterol (mg/dl)	90 ± 29	96 ± 27	87 ± 30	0.48
Body mass index (Kg/m^2)	28 ± 5	29 ± 7	28 ± 3	0.70
Prior LVAD	3 (12%)	2 (22%)	1 (6%)	0.60
Corticosteroid therapy	5 (24%)	4 (44%)	1 (6%)	0.097
Heart weight (g)				
Men	490 ± 58	491 ± 80	492 ± 51	0.91
Women	423 ± 86	438 ± 141	418 ± 71	0.75
Floating heart	12 (48%)	4 (44%)	8 (53%)	1.00

LDL = low density lipoprotein; LVAD =left ventricular assist device.

Discussion

The present report describes 25 patients who underwent OHT because of chronic severe heart failure resulting from cardiac sarcoidosis: 16 of the patients had classic non-caseating granulomas in the operatively-excised native hearts and 9 had no granulomas in the explanted hearts, although 3 of them had typical granulomas in percutaneous biopsies of heart or in the "left ventricular core" excised at the time of insertion of left ventricular assist device. Comparison of various clinical and gross morphologic features of the 16 patients with granulomas in the explanted hearts to the 9 patients without disclosed no significant differences.

Typical gross and histologic features of cardiac sarcoidosis severe enough to warrant OHT include focal but extensive scars in the walls of both left and right ventricles and ventricular septum.[1–8] Scars in the atrial walls are infrequent.[5] The focal scars in the right ventricular wall are usually transmural; those involving the left ventricular wall may also be transmural but often they are only subepicardial, the opposite of what occurs in hearts of patients with coronary heart disease, which is subendocardial or transmural or both but not subepicardial.[9] The ventricular walls are more often thinner than normal rather than thicker than normal. The ventricular cavities are severely dilated (unless a left ventricular assist device had been inserted earlier). Histologically, the non-caseating granulomas are typically located within the scars and numerous ones are present in some scars. In most patients some ventricular wall scars contain granulomas and others do not. The numbers of nuclei present in the giant cells may exceed 50. Lymphocytes also are present.

How can we be certain that the 9 patients without non-caseating granulomas in the explanted hearts have cardiac sarcoidosis? In 3 of these 9 patients an earlier percutaneous biopsy (in 2) or examination of the portion of left ventricular wall excised to insert a left ventricular assist device (in 1) did indeed contain non-caseating granulomas. The interval from this tissue examination to the OHT in these 3 patients was 0.1, 7, and 53 months, respectively. Another supporting factor was that many of the ventricular wall scars in the 16 patients with granulomas present in the explanted heart also had ventricular-wall scars without any granulomas. The latter observation suggests it would not be a "stretch" for all the scars to eventually be devoid of granulomas. Three of the 9 patients without granulomas in the explanted hearts were treated with cortico-steroid therapy, a known cause of converting non-caseating granulomas into scars without granulomas.[1] (Each of the 3 patients in whom the diagnosis was made by examination of cardiac tissue some time before the OHT were treated with prednisone.)

The positive features of this report are the following: (1) no previous report has emphasized that cardiac sarcoidosis may be present without non-caseating granulomas being present in the heart. (2) No previous study has compared clinical and gross morphologic findings in the patients with to those without non-caseating granulomas in the heart.

Limitations of the present study include the following: (1) perhaps not enough histologic sections of myocardium were studied. (We examined at least 4 large

Table 2
Pertinent clinical and morphological findings in 25 patients who had orthotopic heart transplantation for cardiac sarcoidosis

Case	Age (years)	Sex	Race	Duration of symptoms before OHT (months)	BMI I(Kg/m^2)	TC (mg/dl)	LDL (mg/dl)	CI (l/min/m^2)	P-Rx	Clinical cardiac diagnosis	ICD	HW (g)	Heart floats	G	Location of granulomas		
															RV	VS	LV
1	50	F	B	132	25	124	74	–	0	IDC	+	440	0	+	1+	3+	3+
2	52	M	W	192	28	172	108	1.6	+	IDC*	0	440	0	+	1+	2+	1+
3	52	F	B	50	31	166	64	2.3	0	IDC	+	440	0	+	1+	3+	3+
4	53	M	W	12	27	188	112	1.6	0	IDC	0	555	+	+	3+	3+	3+
5	54	F	W	46	26	74	46	1.8	0	IDC	0	425	0	+	3+	3+	3+
6	54	M	W	108	30	210	134	-	0	IDC	0	511	-	+	3+	3+	3+
7	56	F	W	11	26	143	118	–	0	IDC	0	450	+	+	1+	3+	3+
8	57	F	W	46	30	138	94	1.4	0	IDC	0	380	0	+	3+	3+	3+
9	58	F	W	60	27	229	147	2.2	0	IDC	+	560	+	+	3+	3+	3+
10	58	M	W	48	25	114	64	1.2	0	IDC	0	420	0	+	3+	3+	3+
11	59	F	B	72	26	134	69	1.3	0	IDC	+	370	0	+	1+	2+	1+
12	60	F	W	36	28	130	93	1.2	0	IDC	0	401	+	+	1+	3+	3+
13	61	F	W	120	25	119	60	1.2	0	IDC	0	300	+	+	3+	3+	3+
14	63	M	W	84	33	109	52	1.6	0	IDC	+	470	+	+	3+	3+	3+
15	63	M	W	48	24	157	86	1.7	0	IDC	0	540	+	+	3+	3+	3+
16	67	M	W	48	30	116	70	1.6	0	IDC	0	510	+	+	3+	3+	3+
17	40	F	W	11	45	107	78	1.4	0	IDC	0	370	0	0	0	0	0
18	50	M	W	36	28	185	119	1.7	+	CS	+	605	0	0	0	0	0
19	53	M	W	60	31	233	120	1.9	+	CS	0	535	0	0	0	0	0
20	54	F	B	100	24	191	108	1.8	0	IDC	0	345	0	0	0	0	0
21	57	M	W	36	30	119	82	1.2	0	IDC	0	420	+	0	0	0	0
22	59	M	W	48	28	–	–	–	+	CS	+	420	+	0	0	0	0
23	62	F	B	216	19	182	129	1.5	0	IDC	+	600	0	0	0	0	0
24	65	M	B	139	29	160	82	–	+	IDC	+	475	+	0	0	0	0
25	69	M	W	36	23	101	50	1.3	0	IDC	0	475	+	0	0	0	0

AB = black; BMI = body mass index; CI = cardiac index; CS = cardiac sarcoidosis; F = female; G = granuloma; HW = heart weight; I = indirect; ICD = intracardiac defibrillator; IDC = ischemic dilated cardiomyopathy; L = left; LDL = low-density lipoprotein; LV = left ventricle; M = male; OHT = orthotopic heart transplant; P = prednisone Rx; R = right; RV = right ventricle; TC = total cholesterol; VS = ventricular septum; W = white.

* Because the patient had biopsy-proven pulmonary sarcoid, the patient clinically was considered to have cardiac sarcoid as well, but a cardiac biopsy done before the OHT was negative for sarcoid.

Table 3
Electrocardiographic findings before orthotopic heart transplantation in 25 patients with cardiac sarcoidosis

Case	Paced	QRS amplitude in each electrocardiographic lead (mm)												Total 12-lead QRS voltage (mm)	Arrhythmias		BBB (Type)	CHB	Prolonged QT Interval
		I	II	III	aVR	aVL	aVF	V1	V2	V3	V4	V5	V6		A (Type)	V (Type)			
	0	0	0	0	0	0	0	0	0	0	0	0	0	0	0	0			
1	+	2	23	13	6	7	28	4	12	16	20	18	12	161	0	0	+ (NS)	+	0
2	0	14	12	8	13	11	7	12	8	8	18	22	22	155	0	0	+ (R)	0	0
3	+	5	5	5	5	2	8	6	7	7	5	5	7	67	0	+ (VPC)	+ (L)	0	0
4	+	4	12	9	6	3	9	7	7	3	7	10	9	86	0	+ (VPC)	+ (R)	+	0
5	+	4	4	5	2	8	4	–	–	–	–	–	–	–	0	0	0	+	0
6	–	–	–	–	–	–	–	–	–	–	–	–	–	–	–	–	–	-	-
7	+	4	7	8	5	6	8	4	8	4	5	7	7	73	0	+ (VT)	0	0	0
8	0	5	1	6	3	6	4	5	9	5	4	2	2	52	+ (AT)	0	+ (R)	0	0
9	0	8	8	15	3	11	12	5	7	4	4	6	6	89	0	0			
	+	3	3	4	2	3	3	3	7	3	3	4	4	69	0	0	+ (R)	0	0
10	+	9	9	6	4	4	6	5	3	8	8	8	7	77	0	0	+ (L)	0	0
11	0	11	11	17	8	14	13	9	5	9	12	16	19	144	0	0			
	+	10	12	19	8	14	15	8	9	10	13	15	14	147	0	0	+ (R)	+	0
12	0	5	3	4	5	7	3	3	7	4	6	2	5	54	+ (AF)	+ (VPC)	0	0	0
13	+	4	4	5	3	6	4	4	10	5	7	7	8	72	0	0	+ (R)	+	+
14	+	5	12	8	8	5	10	8	9	14	10	9	5	103	0	+ (VPC)	+ (L)	+	0
15	0	8	6	3	6	6	4	9	10	13	18	22	29	134					
	+	5	8	11	5	6	11	2	4	12	17	11	3	95	+ (AF)	+ (VPC)	+ (R)	0	0
16	+	4	5	7	2	5	5	2	2	6	5	3	1	47	0	+ (VT)	+ (NS)	+	0
17	0	18	6	13	6	13	7	6	6	6	6	5	6	98	+ (APC)	+ (VPC)	0	0	0
18	0	7	11	14	5	9	12	6	14	19	7	10	7	121	+ (APC)	0	+ (L)	0	0
19	+	7	7	10	4	8	9	5	7	5	6	7	6	81	0	0	0	+	0
20	0	3	7	7	4	4	6	4	8	11	9	12	14	89	0	0	0	0	+
21	0	5	8	4	5	4	6	7	10	28	26	22	6	131	+ (APC)	0	+ (R)	0	+
22	0	4	1	5	4	3	4	–	–	–	–	–	–	–	0	0	0	0	0
23	0	10	11	10	7	7	7	10	9	7	9	10	10	107	0	0	+ (R)	0	0
24	0	5	7	5	6	4	5	5	4	5	7	10	11	74	+ (AF)	0	+ (R)	0	0
25	0	10	5	6	6	11	12	11	6	4	4	12	4	91	0	0	0	0	0

A = atrial; AF = atrial fibrillation; APC = atrial premature complexes; AT= atrial tachycardia; BBB = bundle branch block; CHB = complete heart block; L = left; NS = non-specific; R = right; V= ventricular; VPC = ventricular premature complexes; VT = ventricular tachycardia.

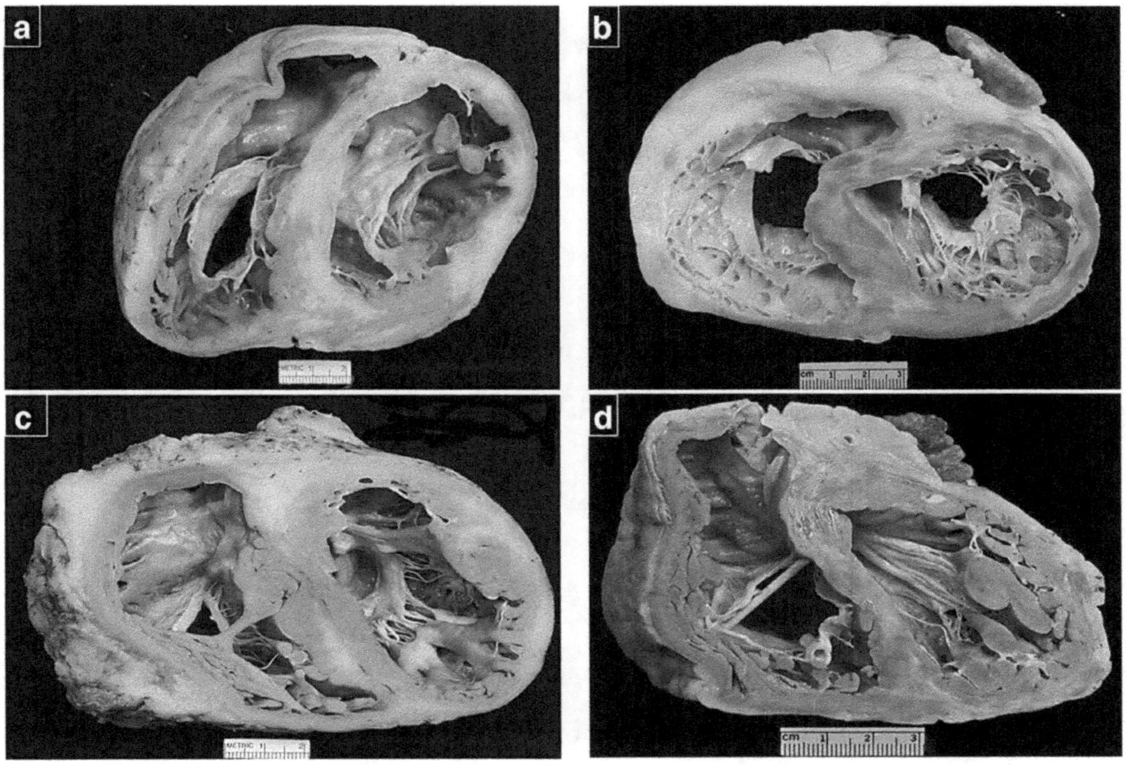

Figure 1. Shown here are basal portions of the heart in 4 patients, 2 of whom (*a* and *c*) had granulomas in the explanted heart and 2, (*b* and *d*) did not. (*a*) patient #5 (Table 2); (*b*) patient #23 (Table 2); (*c*) patient #12 (Table 2); *d*) patient #20 (Table 2). Both ventricles are dilated in each of these 4 patients. Portions of the tricuspid and mitral valves are visible in all 4 patients. The white areas of right ventricular free wall, ventricular septum and left ventricular free wall represent sites of scarring, some of which contained non-caseating granulomas and some of which did not.

[endocardium-to-epicardium] sections of the ventricular walls in all 25 patients and far more [up to 20] in a few patients.); (2) perhaps the 9 patients without tissue proof of cardiac sarcoidosis *in the explanted hearts*, namely the presence of non-caseating granulomas, did not have cardiac sarcoidosis. We believe this scenario to be highly unlikely because 3 of the 9 patients had earlier proof of cardiac sarcoidosis (biopsy or left ventricular "core" examination), and, additionally, we know of no other cardiac condition that even remotely resembles the full-blown morphologic features of cardiac sarcoidosis (Figures 1 and 2).

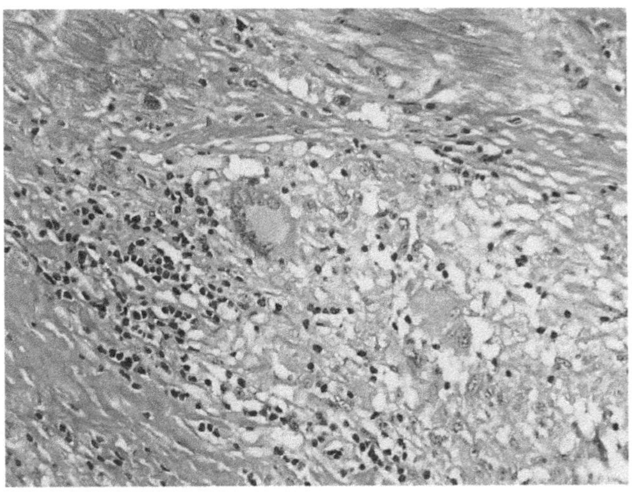

Figure 2. Photomicrograph of a portion of left ventricular free wall in patient #16 (Table 2). The myocardial wall is partially replaced by a dense fibrous tissue which stains blue within which is a sarcoid granuloma. Trichrome stain, original magnification × 40.

1. Roberts WC, McAllister HA Jr, Ferrans VJ. Sarcoidosis of the heart. A clinicopathologic study of 35 necropsy patients (Group I) and review of 78 previously described necropsy patients (Group II). *Am J Med* 1977;63:86–108.
2. Virmani R, Bures JC, Roberts WC. Cardiac sarcoidosis: a major cause of sudden death in young individuals. *Chest* 1980;77:423–428.
3. Donsky AS, Escobar J, Capehart J, Roberts WC. Heart transplantation for undiagnosed cardiac sarcoidosis. *Am J Cardiol* 2002;89:1447–1450.
4. Roberts WC, Vowels TJ, Ko JM, Capehart JE, Hall SA. Cardiac transplantation for cardiac sarcoidosis with initial diagnosis by examination of the left ventricular apical "core" excised for insertion of a left ventricular assist device for severe chronic heart failure. *Am J Cardiol* 2009;103:110–114.
5. Sharma PS, Lubahn JG, Donsky AS, Yoon ADH, Carry MM, Grayburn PA, Wood PB, Ko JM, Burton EC, Roberts WC. Diagnosing cardiac sarcoidosis clinically without tissue confirmation. *Proc (Bayl Univ Med Cent)* 2009;22:236–238.
6. Roberts WC, Chung MS, Ko JM, Capehart JE, Hall SA. Morphologic features of cardiac sarcoidosis in native hearts of patients having cardiac transplantation. *Am J Cardiol* 2014;113:706–712.
7. Armstrong D, Gonzalez-Stawinski GV, Ko JM, Hall SA, Roberts WC. The two extremes of cardiac sarcoidosis and the effect of prednisone therapy. *Am J Cardiol* 2015;115:150–153.
8. Roberts WC, Becker TM, Hall SA. Usefulness of total 12-lead QRS voltage as a clue to diagnosis of patients with cardiac sarcoidosis severe enough to warrant orthotopic heart transplant. *JAMA Cardiol* 2018;3:64–68.
9. Shirani J, Roberts WC. Subepicardial myocardial lesions. *Am Heart J* 1993;125:1346–1352.

www.ingramcontent.com/pod-product-compliance
Lightning Source LLC
LaVergne TN
LVHW062150200926
848484LV00007B/1894
9798886800883